ANNUAL REVIEW OF NURSING RESEARCH

Volume 10, 1992

ANNUAL REVIEW OF NURSING RESEARCH

Volume 10

Joyce J. Fitzpatrick, Ph.D.
Roma Lee Taunton, Ph.D.
Ada K. Jacox, Ph.D.
Editors

SPRINGER PUBLISHING COMPANY
New York

Order ANNUAL REVIEW OF NURSING RESEARCH, Volume 10, 1992, prior to publication and receive a 10% discount. An order coupon can be found at the back of this volume.

Springer Publishing Company, Inc.
536 Broadway
New York, NY 10012

92 93 94 95 96 / 5 4 3 2 1

ISBN-0-8261-4359-8
ISSN-0739-6686

ANNUAL REVIEW OF NURSING RESEARCH is indexed in *Cumulative Index to Nursing and Allied Health Literature and Index Medicus*.

Printed in the United States of America

Contents

PREFACE

Publication of this tenth volume of the *Annual Review of Nursing Research* (ARNR) series represents an important milestone for the scientific nursing community as we enter our second decade of publication. We have witnessed the expansion in the number of nurse researchers, a healthy increase in the amount of public and private funding for nursing research and, most importantly, a significant increase in the number and quality of scholarly publications in nursing.

In this special tenth volume, Joanne Sabol Stevenson recounts the history of the *Annual Review of Nursing Research* series and examines the reviews. This introductory chapter will undoubtedly go down in history, for Stevenson captures not only the content of the series, but also the spirit of its authors and editors. We recognize her unique contribution to the current volume.

Our tenth volume would not be complete without recognition of the significant contributions of a number of individuals. The *ARNR* Advisory Board members have served us well over the first 10 years. We extend a special thank you to Jeanne Quint Benoliol, Doris Block, Ellen Fuller, Susan Gortner, Ada Sue Hinshaw, Ada Jacox, Janelle Krueger, Angela McBride, Joanne Stevenson, Harriet Werley, and Margaret Williams, our Advisory Board Members. Rosemary Ellis and Lucille Notter also served as Board members. Our Board members have provided advice, critiqued manuscripts, brainstormed about future volumes, and recommended countless reviewers, topics, and authors. We recognize their long-term commitment to this project. Second, we have been fortunate to have a series of editors, all of whom brought special talents to this project. First and foremost, tribute is paid to our founding editor, Harriet H. Werley. And an unending thank you to our subsequent editors Roma Lee Taunton, coeditor of volumes four through ten, Jeanne Quint Benoliol, coeditor of volumes six through eight, and Ada Jacox, coeditor of volumes nine and ten. Nikki Polis, who joined the editorial staff with volume four, has provided an important consistency to our project. Her efforts on behalf of this *ARNR* series should be noted and heralded in our history.

In selecting topics for this volume, we included aspects of nursing research that were currently of high priority. As in previous volumes, there is a theme for Part I. In this volume, the theme of current critical nursing problems has been selected for the practice section. Thus, in the Nursing Practice section, we have included the following chapters: urinary incontinence in older adults by Kathleen A. McCormick and Mary Palmer, diabetes mellitus research by Edna Hamera; research on battered women and their children by Jacquelyn C. Campbell and Barbara Parker; chronic mental illness research by Jeanne C. Fox; and research on childhood and adolescent bereavement by Nancy D. Opie. In the section on Nursing Care Delivery, Susan Riesch reviews research on nursing centers and in the Nursing Education section, Ruth A. Anderson reviews research on nursing administration education. The Profession section includes two chapters: reviews of alcohol and drug abuse among nurses by Eleanor J. Sullivan and Sandra M. Handley and research on the hospital staff nurse role by Norma L. Chaska. In the final section, Beverly M. Henry and Jean M. Nagelkerk review international nursing research.

In recognition of the conclusion of our first decade and the publication of this tenth volume, a special International State of the Science Congress is being held in August, 1992, in Washington, DC. Nurse leaders in science development, education, management, and clinical practice will join together to celebrate our accomplishments in this past decade. Over 200 scientific papers will be delivered by nurses from this country and abroad. Further, authors of key invited papers for the plenary sessions will provide exemplars of the significant strides in nursing research in their chosen area. With more than 10 national and regional nursing organizations cosponsoring this conference, nurses' scientific contributions will be acknowledged from a broad range of participants. Further, invited papers delivered at the conference will be compiled in a special tenth year anniversary supplement to the *Annual Review of Nursing Research* series. We look forward to your participation at this important conference and hope that you join us in the continued celebration.

JOYCE J. FITZPATRICK
EDITOR

Contributors

Ruth A. Anderson, Ph.D.
School of Nursing
University of Texas at Austin
Austin, Texas

Jacquelyn C. Campbell, Ph.D.
College of Nursing
Wayne State University
Detroit, Michigan

Norma L. Chaska, Ph.D.
School of Nursing
University of San Francisco
San Francisco, California

Jeanne C. Fox, Ph.D.
School of Nursing
University of Virginia
Charlottesville, Virginia

Edna Hamera, Ph.D.
School of Nursing
University of Kansas Medical Center
Kansas City, Kansas

Sandra M. Handley, Ph.D.
School of Nursing
University of Kansas Medical Center
Kansas City, Kansas

Beverly M. Henry, Ph.D.
College of Nursing
University of Illinois at Chicago
Chicago, Illinois

Kathleen A. McCormick, Ph.D.
Office of the Forum
for Quality and Effectiveness
in Health Care,
Agency for
Health Care Policy and Research
(AHCPR)
Rockville, Maryland

Jean M. Nagelkerk, Ph.D.
Department of Nursing
University of Tampa
Tampa, Florida

Nancy D. Opie, DNS
College of Nursing and Health
University of Cincinnati
Cincinnati, Ohio

Mary H. Palmer, Ph.D.
National Institutes of Health
National Institute on Aging
Gerontology Research Center
Baltimore, Maryland

Barbara Parker, Ph.D.
School of Nursing
University of Maryland
Baltimore, Maryland

Susan K. Riesch, DNSc
School of Nursing
University of Wisconsin-Milwaukee
Milwaukee, Wisconsin

Joanne Sabol Stevenson, Ph.D.
Professor, Department of
Life Span Process
The Ohio State University
Columbus, Ohio

Eleanor J. Sullivan
School of Nursing
University of Kansas
Lawrence, Kansas

FORTHCOMING

ANNUAL REVIEW OF NURSING RESEARCH, Volume 11

Tentative Contents

Chapter 1

Review of the First Decade of the *Annual Review of Nursing Research*

JOANNE SABOL STEVENSON
COLLEGE OF NURSING
THE OHIO STATE UNIVERSITY

CONTENTS

An annual review of literature can have utilitarian value for its consumers in at least three ways: (a) it makes conducting literature reviews more efficient because a foundation is given from which to build or pursue a point of departure; (b) recommendations for future research contained in the reviews can give guidance to graduate students and others who are building a program of research; and (c) in the policy arena critical reviews can have an impact at many levels. Examples of public policy uses of reviews include: decisions to make a research topic a public sector priority for support; decision by a (nursing) specialty group to incorporate research findings into standards of care or other forms of utilization, decisions by educators to include a body of findings in the curriculum, or decisions by legislators to approve third-party coverage for a (nursing) intervention based on the results of research.

Harriet Werley had a dream of developing an annual integrative critical review of published nursing research. She already had a number of innovations to her credit: the first clinical nursing research center at the Walter Reed Army Institute of Research in 1957; the first interdisciplinary health research center at Wayne State University in 1969; the publication of *Research in Nursing and Health* in 1978—the second journal of nursing research, but the first with an entrepreneurial publisher (John Wiley & Sons); and the gathering of all the research development academics in the Midwest. The latter effort led to her Division of Nursing federally funded project entitled "Nurse Faculty Research Development in the Midwest," which served as the springboard for the Midwest Nursing Research Society (Stevenson, 1987). By 1980 Werley had garnered considerable support for the annual review series. She pursued the idea relentlessly with informal "advisory" group consultations during national and regional meetings. During this early planning stage, she received a vote of support for the new series during a membership meeting of the American Nurses Association Council of Nurse Researchers.

In 1982 Dr. Ursula Springer, President of the Springer Publishing Company, took a significant risk in agreeing to publish the proposed *Annual Review of Nursing Research (ARNR)* series. No one could prove that there was an adequate amount of research being published on any one topic of nursing research to justify an annual review. However, both editor and publisher believed an annual review series could serve as a stimulus for more research in the maturing discipline. There was evidence, such as the growing number of nurses with earned doctorates who could do research and growing number of master's-prepared clinicians and managers who could comprehend and use results of research, that nursing was a profession on the rise.

INITIATING THE *ARNR* SERIES

In the 36 months before the first volume of the *ARNR* went to press, many activities related to setting the standards for reviews, commissioning chapters, and related work occurred simultaneously. Writing for the annual review series was unlike any experience heretofore experienced by most nurse scholars. Guidelines were developed that might have been assumed in more mature fields but were important to specify for the state-of-nursing research at that time. The invited authors were to be senior nurse scholars, the inclusion of students or nonresearchers as co-authors was discouraged, and unpublished works such as master's theses or unpublished doctoral dissertations generally were to be excluded. The series was to be critical review of *published* research that would serve as a springboard for setting further research directions in each topic area.

The planning for the first three volumes went on at the same time in order to create a timeline that would permit about 3 years of progressive deadlines for authors and reviewers, including several months for the publication process. Volume 1 was the 1983 volume but it actually carries a copyright date of 1984. After Volume 1 the year in which the volume was published has been consistent with the copyright year.

Established researchers were given the responsibility for doing critical reviews with the intent that these reviewers would possess a sense of experiential history and wisdom, a longer term perspective of progress in the content area of the review, a track record of research and scholarship, and a set of connections to the invisible college of colleagues to find the elusive publications whose titles do not permit access through computerized searches. Another important goal of inviting reputable scholars with track records was to ensure high-quality reviews and to enhance the probability that scholars in other health fields would also come to value and use the material in the series (H. Werley, personal communication, 1991).

Development of the guidelines and directions to authors was aided by Werley's previous experience with an annual review in another field and Springer's experience with the *Annual Review of Gerontology*. The purpose of the guidelines was to encourage a balanced critical review of the literature. The 1982 article by Cooper on integrative research reviews became a routine part of the *ARNR* guideline packet; it has been helpful in guiding authors to be analytical and critical rather than simply doing cataloguing or summarizing.

During the months of preliminary discussions with many nursing groups, there were numerous discussions about how to divide the volumes into chapters. Considerations included the important areas of nursing research that would inform the field, choosing areas where there was a corpus of studies to review, and a category system that fit nursing rather than the conceptualizations of other disciplines (H. Werley, personal communication, 1991). From these discussions evolved the outline of chapters that has been used during the first decade of volumes.

From the beginning, the journal was organized with the largest set of chapters (usually five) on a theme related to nursing practice. The next three sections of reviews were devoted to research on nursing care delivery, nursing education, and the profession of nursing. The final section was called "Other" and included reviews on philosophic inquiry (Ellis, 1984), international nursing research, and other special topics. Werley wanted one chapter in each volume from outside the United States, but scheduling and other difficulties got in the way and the first such chapter was included in Volume 2.

The decision to devote five chapters to nursing practice and fewer chapters to the other topics reflected the trend of the 1970s to move away from an emphasis on nursing education research and research on nurses in favor of nursing practice research. This trend had been emphasized by the various groups of nurse-researchers with whom Werley consulted in the late 1970s.

The nursing practice section has been the mainstay of the series through the years, but it is also the section that has involved the most ambiguity for authors and editors alike. In 1980 the field did not have consensus on a definition of nursing (practice) research that could provide operational guidelines for reviewers about what was and what was not appropriate material to review for this journal. The alternate interpretations that reviewers might embrace about nursing research were: (a) any research as long as it was *conducted by nurses,* (b) research on a topic in the nursing domain but only involving that corpus of *studies done by nurses,* (c) *a specific content topic* of scientific inquiry regardless of who did the investigations, or (d) *a special way of looking* at a health-related problem from a *nursing* perspective.

There were two ramifications for the series of this definitional ambiguity. The most frequently asked questions of the editors by the authors has been "What do you mean by nursing research?" and "What literature should I review for my chapter?" Obvious options were to review: (a) only work appearing in nursing journals, (b) work published anywhere but with a nurse author or co-author, (c) background theory and research from other fields but culminating with research by nurses, or (d) all work on a topic of particular interest to knowledge development in nursing. This latter definition would mean that the research question or phenomenon was within the purview or responsibility of nursing but very important components of the body of literature (theories, basic science studies, and/or clinical studies) existed in the broader literature.

ARNR reviewers chose a variety of approaches to resolve the dilemma of defining nursing research. Some of this variation will be described later in this chapter for it led to significant variability in the comprehensiveness and utility of the chapters contained in the first 10 volumes.

Werley actually provided a fairly clear sense of her definition of nursing research when she wrote in the preface to Volume 1 "in the judgment of the senior editor of this newly created medium, a review should be limited to research pertinent to nursing and health, and should result in a systematic assessment of knowledge development. Thus it would . . . provide nursing with an appropriate data-based foundation" (Werley, 1984, p. vii). It is interesting to note that she did not imply that the review should be limited to research conducted by nurses. Her statement implies any research as long as it is "pertinent" to nursing and health and "provides nursing with an appropriate . . . foundation." Hence, it is interesting that the overwhelming majority of authors over the subsequent 10 years reviewed only studies with nurses as sole or co-authors. The definitions of nursing research that were used in the vast majority of chapters in the 10 volumes seem to have been: (a) research on a topic pertinent to nursing and (b) limited to that corpus of studies conducted by nurses or including at least one nurse co-investigator.

LEADERSHIP FOR THE FIRST 10 VOLUMES

Werley chose Joyce Fitzpatrick to be the first co-editor. The original Advisory Board members were: Jeanne Quint Benoliel, Doris Bloch, Ellen Fuller, Susan Gortner, Ada Sue Hinshaw, Ada Jacox, Janelle Krueger, Angela Barron McBride, Lucille Notter, Joanne Stevenson, and Margaret Williams. Rosemary Ellis was added a year later, but became terminally ill shortly thereafter. This board represented a mix of clinical expertise and research foci; all members had considerable experience with research development in nursing.

The first change in editors occurred in Volume 4 (1986) when Roma Lee Taunton became a co-editor. Taunton had been a doctoral student and Werley's research assistant during the planning and early development of the *ARNR* series. At the end of work on Volume 4, Werley retired as senior editor and became a member of the Advisory Board. So the Volume 5 co-editors were Fitzpatrick and Taunton. For Volume 6 the editorial team was expanded to include Fitzpatrick, Taunton, and Jeanne Quint Benoliel: Ada Jacox became a co-editor for Volumes 9 and 10 with Fitzpatrick and Taunton.

The makeup of the editorial teams and the Board is indicative of Werley's philosophy and style. She started her projects with a more junior colleague as the second-in-command, intending to turn over the reigns in a few years. It was also her style to choose senior persons for the role of advisors to her projects.

THE FIRST 4 VOLUMES: SETTING THE PRECEDENTS

The themes of the nursing practice sections for the first 3 volumes of the series were planned together. The themes were life-span developmental research for Volume 1, family research for Volume 2, and community research for Volume 3. These three research foci were consensually important to nursing practice. The life-span developmental theme was chosen for Volume 1 because it was believed that this was the most prolific area of published nursing research. Chapters were devoted to each age group and culminated with a review by Jean Quint Benoliel of the death and dying research.

The section on nursing care delivery in Volume 1 included a review of the work on nurse turnover, stress, and satisfaction by Ada Sue Hinshaw and Janet Atwood and a review by Janelle Krueger on interorganizational relations research. The final two chapters were focused on roles in nursing by Mary Conway and philosophic inquiry by Rosemary Ellis. All the chapters in this volume were broad; the average number of citations per chapter was over 80 and the average number of subcategories of each topic was six. This broadness of topics was reflective of the early stage of evolution of nursing research at that time.

It is interesting to note that a few guidelines for authors were not adhered to from the onset of the series. Kathryn Barnard in Chapter 1 and Joanne Stevenson in Chapter 3 of Volume 1 cited several doctoral dissertations; Barnard even used master's theses. The editors accepted the judgments of the authors that the reviews were strengthened by the addition of these unpublished works. The field was still young and some of the important seminal work was being done by graduate students as the offshoot of studies by their mentors. This was particularly true in parent–child nursing, where graduate students did spin-off studies focused on research questions generated through the work of senior investigators.

In four of the first five chapters in the nursing practice section, authors reviewed only studies conducted by nurse-researchers. In contrast, Benoliel's review of research on death, dying, and terminal illness included integration of selected components of the extensive work of nonnurse thanatologists, in addition to the studies by nurses. It provided a fairly comprehensive review of the topic on death and dying focused on those components of particular interest to nursing. Benoliel thus set a precedent for comprehensive reviews on a topic wherein all relevant work, on the components of interest to nursing, was reviewed regardless of the disciplinary background of the investigators.

The decision to employ a developmental model for Volume 1 had mixed results. The area of infants and young children (Bernard's review) had the most published and unpublished work. The nursing research related to schoolagers and adolescents reviewed by Mary Denyes included fewer studies but still a notable amount. However, in the review of research on adults, very few relevant studies were found in the literature. The review on adults by Stevenson was focused on areas where research on adult development might be expected but was not found. This chapter was commissioned by the editors with the goal of reviewing what was published and then using some space to lay out a plan for future research in the area. That was done through the inclusion of a model for future nursing research on adulthood. The chapter on older adults by Mary Opal Wolanin was comprised of studies of ill elders;

thus it did not adhere to the life-span developmental perspective of the first three chapters in this volume. It contained mostly descriptive studies by nurses about symptoms and conditions in late life. Wolanin noted that there were very few intervention studies in the literature at that time.

Volume 2 (1984) contained some chapters in the nursing practice section that were narrower in scope than any of the ones in Volume 1. Regina Lederman did a review on anxiety and conflict during pregnancy; Angela Barron McBride's was on the experience of being a parent; and Jean Johnson reviewed the studies on coping with elective surgery. By narrowing their topics, these authors were able to present more comprehensive reviews of the topics.

Many of Lederman's citations were from outside nursing, and this afforded a more comprehensive synthesis of the state of the art on her topic than would have been possible from the nurse-produced research alone. Lederman's approach was thus somewhat akin to Benoliel's in Volume 1. In addition, Lederman's narrower topic allowed her to focus on her particular area of expertise, such that her judgments about the state of knowledge were firmly grounded from her own program of research.

The section on Nursing Education Research made its first appearance in Volume 2 with three chapters. The topics were teaching-learning (Rheba De Tornyay), students (Patricia Schwirian), and curriculum (Marilyn Stember). Nursing education research chapters had been commissioned for Volume 1, but it took time to receive the first completed chapters.

Werley's goal to include international nursing research also came to fruition in Volume 2. The first such review was developed by Lisbeth Hockey and Margaret Clark on nursing research in Scotland.

As planned, Volume 3 was focused on community-related research. Grayce Sills and Jean Goeppinger presented a general chapter on the community-related research done by nurses. Other reviews in this volume included work on school nursing (Shu-Pi Chen and Judith Sullivan) wherein the reviewers stated that 50% of the citations had no nurse as author. The review of cross-cultural studies (Toni Tripp-Reimer and Molly Dougherty) included only studies by nurses. Ramona Mercer identified her topic of teenage pregnancy as a complex interdisciplinary problem; her solution was to review every study where a nurse was either the sole author or one of a group of authors. She also reviewed studies from journals outside nursing. Thus she cast a somewhat larger net compared to many other reviewers.

The nursing practice chapters in Volume 3 were unique in that only teenage pregnancy was about a concrete health problem. The review on school nursing was akin to ones in other volumes on nursing care delivery. The one on cross-cultural nursing cast a broad net that included several practice-oriented topics such as research on caring, health beliefs, and cross-cultural health practices. It also gave considerable attention to the theories, methods, and values underlying cross-cultural research.

The section on nursing care delivery included a review of studies of nurse practitioners (Sherry Shamansky), which not surprisingly consisted of studies of their acceptance and their impact. An early review of literature on nursing diagnosis by Marjory Gordon turned up only a small number of studies at that time. The section on education was focused on continuing education (Alice Kuramoto) and doctoral education (Juanita Murphy) of nurses; and the section on the profession included ethical inquiry (Susan Gortner) and nursing cost-effectiveness analysis (Claire Fagin and Barbara Jacobsen). The studies of cost-effectiveness were focused on studies of organizational alternatives, such as primary nursing or all-registered nursing (RN) staffs, on alternatives to institutionalization, such as home care, and on nursing care delivery models as care interventions.

In the section on other research, Frederick Suppe and Ada Jacox reviewed the philosophy of science literature. While the work of nurses was featured, the backdrop was the state of knowledge in the general philosophy of science literature. Volume 3 had two nonnurse authors (Jacobsen and Suppe). Their participation extended the expertise in the conduct and interpretation of the specific chapters. Jacobsen had experience in cost studies and Suppe was a well regarded scholar of history and philosophy.

During her doctoral work and later, Werley had studied the editorial processes and decisions of the *Annual Review of Psychology (ARP)* (H. Werley, personal communication, 1991). She believed the *ARP* model of repeating topics in subsequent volumes was a useful idea since it allowed updating of research in fast growing areas of research. This approach was also efficient for doctoral students and others seeking an overview of developments in targeted areas in advance of their own in-depth review of the literature.

Thus it was not surprising that the Nursing Practice Section of Volume 4 featured a return to the life-span development model of Volume 1. This time, however, some of the reviews were on more narrowly focused topics within each age grouping; one example was a second chapter, by Lederman. She reviewed the literature on the effects of maternal anxiety during pregnancy on fetal and newborn health status. The review on a topic in middle adulthood was prepared by Ann Voda and Theresa George; they critiqued the work on menopause. For the review on older adulthood, Mary Adams expanded and updated Wolanin's review from Volume 1. Adams used a different category system and expanded some components of the topic. Most notably, she put more emphasis on activities of daily living, enhancing self-esteem, and optimizing care environments and less on negative consequences of aging. Finally, the death and dying chapter by Alice Demi and Margaret Miles was on bereavement, including studies clustered into parental grief after losing a child, grief of children, and grief among the widowed.

The form and style of the *ARNR* series was fairly crystallized by the time the fourth volume was published. In the subsequent six volumes, the approaches taken by the early authors were repeated. The majority reviewed only studies authored or co-authored by nurses. There were a few reviewers who narrowed their topics and did more comprehensive reviews of literature. In these instances, generally the topics were narrowed so as to be more pertinent to the domain of nursing, but the corpus of studies reviewed was broadened to include all relevant studies regardless of the disciplinary background of the investigator.

CONTENT FOCI OF THE FIRST 10 VOLUMES

Many topics of interest in nursing were reviewed within the first 10 volumes. A series of tables was constructed to categorize the topics and list the specific chapter topics, authors, and citations. In some instances, a topic fit into more than one category and thus appeared in more than one table.

This categorization of the reviews may be helpful to the nursing community, including graduate students and others who are making choices about foci for programs of research. It may prove useful to faculty in making reading assignments for students. It also could be useful for gleaning topics that have not yet been reviewed but could be targeted for future chapters during the next decade.

Life-Span Developmental Perspective

The first category listing, shown in Table 1.1, is The Life-Span Developmental Perspective. This perspective has been a very strong force in the conduct of studies about nursing care of neonates, children, and, to a lesser extent, adolescents.

Interest in maternal–child, infants', and children's health has been strong and consistent within nursing, and over many years there has been considerable research on pregnancy, the neonatal period, early development, and parenting and care of high-risk newborns. Special topics that provide rich information for both preventive and remedial nursing interventions were included in reviews on the effects of stress during the brain growth spurt by Burns and anxiety in pregnancy and effects of maternal anxiety on fetuses and newborns, both by Lederman. The subtopics covered about schoolagers and adolescents were analogous to the subtopics in the neonatal and infant

Table 1.1 Life-Span Developmental Perspective

Maternal–Child Health, Infants, and Young Children		Volume &
Title	*Author(s)*	*Pages*
Nursing Research Related to Infants and Young Children	Barnard, K. E.	*1,* 3–25
The Effect of Stress During the Brain Growth Spurt	Burns, E. M.	*8,* 57–82
Anxiety and Conflict in Pregnancy: Relationship to Maternal Health Status	Lederman, R. P.	*2,* 27–61
Maternal Anxiety in Pregnancy: Relationship to Fetal and Newborn Health Status	Lederman, R. P.	*4,* 3–19
Nurse-Midwifery Care: 1925 to 1984	Thompson, J. E.	*4,* 153–173
Parent–Child Nursing Education	Alexander, C.	*7,* 157–170

Schoolage Children and Adolescents		Volume &
Title	*Author(s)*	*Pages*
Nursing Research Related to Schoolage Children and Adolescents	Denyes, M. J.	*1,* 27–53
Preschool Children	Fleming, J. W.	*4,* 21–54
Health Promotion and Illness Prevention	Pender, N. J.	*2,* 83–105
Childhood and Adolescent Bereavement	Opie, N.	*10,* 127–141
Teenage Pregnancy as a Community Problem	Mercer, R. M.	*3,* 49–76
School Nursing	Chen, S. C., & Sullivan, J. A.	*3,* 25–48

Adulthood		Volume &
Title	*Author(s)*	*Pages*
Adulthood: A Promising Focus for Future Research	Stevenson, J. S.	*1,* 55–74
Health Promotion and Illness Prevention	Pender, N. J.	*2,* 83–105
Menopause	Voda, A. M., & George, T.	*4,* 55–75

Older Adult Issues and Problems		Volume &
Title	*Author(s)*	*Pages*
Clinical Geriatric Nursing Research	Wolanin, M. O.	*1,* 75–99
Aging: Gerontological Nursing Research	Adams, M.	*4,* 77–103
Arthritis	Lambert, V. A.	*9,* 3–18
Alzheimer's Disease	Maas, M., & Buckwalter, K.	*9,* 19–55
Home Health Care	Barkauskas, V. H.	*8,* 103–132
Family Caregiving for the Elderly	Given, B., & Given, C.	*9,* 77–101

Table 1.1 (*Continued*)

Family Research *Title*	*Author(s)*	*Volume & Pages*
Family Research: Issues and Directions for Nursing	Feetham, S. L.	2, 3–25
The Experience of Being a Parent	McBride, A. B.	2, 63–81
Family Adaptation to a Child's Chronic Illness	Austin, J. K.	9, 103–120
Family Caregiving for the Elderly	Given, B., & Given, C.	9, 77–101

research. Subtopics included in both age groups were optimizing child development, social/familial, and environmental influences on development and health, and research on the experiences and procedures of being ill and hospitalized. Both categories included delivery-oriented chapters (nurse-midwifery and school nursing). Just as the maternal–child health/neonatal/infant section included special topics (nurse-midwifery and school nursing), the schoolagers and adolescents topic included chapters on teenage pregnancy and the effects of bereavement during these developmental stages. The most important outcome that emerged from these studies was the apparent power of nursing practice to improve the outcomes for these patients quite aside from the impact of medical care.

In contrast, the developmental perspective has been almost nonexistent on the care of young, middle, and older adults. Although much research has been devoted to young and middle adults, it has been conducted from an acute-care, long-term care, or rehabilitation focus. Similarly research on the elderly was conducted from a "geriatric" problem-centered orientation and more recently has shifted to functional independence. There has not been much research on normal development and optimizing health during the adult life stages. One complete chapter (Stevenson's) and a portion of the Pender chapter include a direct focus on adult age groups from a developmental perspective. The chapter on menopause by Voda and George could be considered a developmental topic and so it is included in this section of Table 1.1.

There were six chapters devoted to topics relevant to older adults. Besides the ones by Wolanin and Adams, there were some on diseases that affect mostly older adults, such as Alzheimer's disease, and one on family caregiving of older adults.

The last subcategory in Table 1.1 is family research. Five chapters were devoted to family research. Reviews by Feetham and Fleming provided general overviews of all family research of interest to nursing practice. The third was on research related to being a parent (McBride) and the other two were about the family in relation to illness of children (Austin) and as informal caregivers to the elderly (Given and Given). The general finding about this area of research was that there are difficulties related to measuring family phenomena; use of a single respondent is frowned upon, but there is not agreement about what to do instead. Most of the work was focused on characteristics and behaviors of family members and very few intervention studies were found. There seems to be consensus that family research is essential in nursing, but a major breakthrough in methodology is needed.

Clinical Research Topics

The length of Table 1.2 attests to the fact that the largest number of reviews have been on research relevant to nursing practice. The first list shows two chapters on nursing diagnosis research and the rest of the list are on nursing activities, interventions, or therapeutics. The next two lists cover those symptoms and problems frequently faced in nursing practice such as pain, incontinence, physiologic responses of patients, and the physiologic mechanisms and rhythms that are critical to caring for patients. Examples include sleep and other biologic rhythms, information processing, and nutritional status.

Other themes that received considerable attention over the decade were crises, grief, loss, and bereavement. There were seven chapters dedicated to some aspect of these topics, showing the importance to nursing. In these studies researchers attempted to uncover emotions, coping mechanisms, or untoward outcomes operating during these stresses and to find productive approaches to care and intervention.

The final list in Table 1.2 contains topics that are broad and form a basic context for all of nursing practice. The list does not lend itself to easy categorization because it cuts across all areas of practice. Women's health and cross-cultural research are two such topics reviewed in the first decade of the *ARNR*.

Table 1.3 is presented as a separate table. Yet, although most of the topics fit under nursing practice, they are also relevant to nursing care delivery, nursing education, and the profession. These topics are essential to any field. Every discipline and profession must know its history, have a prevailing philosophy, develop and test theories, and engage in moral and ethical behavior. Seven chapters during the decade were devoted to reviews of inquiry on these topics.

Research on Nursing Care Delivery

There were 14 reviews published on various aspects of nursing care delivery. Some were dedicated to the occupational or worker aspects, such as nurse

Table 1.2 Nursing Practice

Nursing Diagnoses and Interventions		
Title	*Author(s)*	*Volume & Pages*
Nursing Diagnosis	Gordon, M.	*3,* 127–146
Nursing Diagnosis	Kim, M. J.	*7,* 117–142
Relaxation	Snyder, M.	*6,* 111–128
Touch	Weiss, S. J.	*6,* 3–27
Patient Contracting	Boehm, S.	*7,* 143–153
Patient Education Part I	Lindeman, C. A.	*6,* 29–60
Patient Education Part II	Lindeman, C. A.	*7,* 199–212
The Physical Environment and Patient Care	Williams, M. A.	*6,* 61–84
Social Support	Norbeck, J. S.	*6,* 85–109
Endotracheal Suctioning	Stone, K. S., & Turner, B.	*7,* 27–49
Prevention of Pressure Sores	Carlson, C. E., & King, R. B.	*8,* 35–56
Infection Control	Larson, E. L.	*7,* 95–113
Interpersonal Communication Between Nurses and Patients	Garvin, B. J., & Kennedy, C. W.	*8,* 213–234

Symptoms and Problems		
Title	*Author(s)*	*Volume & Pages*
Stress	Lyon, B. L., & Werner, J. S.	*5,* 3–22
Physiologic Responses to Stress	Doswell, W. M.	*7,* 51–69
Pain	Taylor, A. G.	*5,* 23–43
Urinary Incontinence in Older Adults	McCormick, K. A., & Palmer, M.	*10,* 25–53
Physiologic Responses in Health and Illness	Kim, M. J.	*5,* 79–104

Risk Behaviors and Forms of Abuse		
Title	*Author(s)*	*Volume & Pages*
Battered Women and Their Children	Campbell, J., & Parker, B.	*10,* 77–94
Smoking Cessation: Research on Relapse Crises	O'Connell, K. A.	*8,* 83–100

Table 1.2 (*Continued*)

Focus on Physiologic Mechanisms and Biologic Rhythms		*Volume &*
Title	*Author(s)*	*Pages*
Human Biologic Rhythms	Felton, G.	*5,* 45–77
Human Information Processing	Roy, C., Sr.	*6,* 237–262
Sleep	Shaver J., & Giblin, E. C.	*7,* 71–93
Nutritional Studies in Nursing	Bodkin, N. L., & Hansen, B. C.	*9,* 203–220

Care Problems of Specific Diseases		*Volume &*
Title	*Author(s)*	*Pages*
Arthritis	Lambert, V. A.	*9,* 3–18
Alzheimer's Disease	Maas, M., & Buckwalter, K.	*9,* 19–55
Chronic Mental Illness	Fox, J.	*10,* 95–112
Diabetes Mellitus	Hamera, E.	*10,* 55–75

Research in Nursing Specialty Areas		*Volume &*
Title	*Author(s)*	*Pages*
School Nursing	Chen, S. C., & Sullivan, J. A.	*3,* 25–48
Nurse-Midwifery Care: 1925 to 1984	Thompson, J. E.	*4,* 153–173
Critical Care Nursing	Dracup, K.	*5,* 107–133
Neurologic Nursing Research	Parson, L. C., & Kidd, P. S.	*7,* 3–25
Cardiovascular Nursing Research	Cowan, M. J.	*8,* 3–33

Crises, Grief, Loss, and Bereavement		*Volume &*
Title	*Author(s)*	*Pages*
Nursing Research on Death, Dying, and Terminal Illness: Development, Present State, and Prospects	Benoliel, J. Q.	*1,* 101–130
Bereavement	Demi, A. S., & Shandor-Miles, M. S.	*4,* 105–123
Coping with Elective Surgery	Johnson, J. E.	*2,* 107–132
Human Responses to Catastrophe	Murphy, S. A.	*9,* 57–76
Family Adaptation to a Child's Chronic Illness	Austin, J. K.	*9,* 103–120
Childhood and Adolescent Bereavement	Opie, N.	*10,* 127–141
Disaster Nursing	Komnenich, P., & Feller, C.	*9,* 123–134

Table 1.2 (*Continued*)

Research on Special Populations		Volume &
Title	*Author(s)*	*Pages*
Women's Health	Woods, N. F.	*6*, 209–236
Cross-Cultural Nursing Research	Tripp-Reimer, T., & Dougherty, M. C.	*3*, 77–104

turnover, stress, and evaluation and measurement of quality of care. Others included reviews of studies of specialty practice, such as critical care nursing, public health nursing, nursing administration, and nurse anesthesia care. A third cluster included reviews on sites of practice, such as nursing centers and home health care. In the list of studies on costs and policy-related research, there were two reviews on cost-related research and one on policy-related research. The review by Turner on acquired immunodeficiency syndrome (AIDS) appears in two tables; it was put in Table 1.4 because some of the studies were about managing the delivery of nursing service to AIDS patients.

Research on Professional Issues

Research on several professional issues was included during the past decade (see Table 1.5). Seven chapters were categorized under this theme. Topics included issues about roles such as the staff nurse role, leadership research, studies of men in nursing, and research on faculty practice. The reviews on acquired immunodeficiency syndrome (AIDS) and drug and alcohol abuse were placed here. The AIDS chapter contains a review of studies about

Table 1.3 Historical, Ethical, Theoretical, and Philosophic Inquiry in Nursing

Title	*Author(s)*	*Volume & Pages*
Nursing's Heritage	Palmer, I. S.	*4*, 237–257
Philosophic Inquiry	Ellis, R.	*1*, 211–228
Philosophy of Science and the Development of Nursing Theory	Suppe, F., & Jacox, A. K.	*3*, 241–267
Ethical Inquiry	Gortner, S. R.	*3*, 193–214
Moral Reasoning and Ethical Practice	Ketefian, S.	*7*, 173–195
Conceptual Models of Nursing	Silva, M. C.	*5*, 229–246
Health Conceptualizations	Newman, M. A.	*9*, 221–243

nurses' attitudes toward AIDS and other professional behavior considerations. The drug and alcohol abuse chapter includes research on addictive disorders in nurses.

Educational Research in Nursing

There were 17 reviews categorized under education (see Table 1.6). Education was viewed as inclusive of basic, advanced/specialty, graduate, postgraduate, and continuing education. It also included teaching strategies, such as computer-aided instruction research, and teaching complex skills, such as clinical judgment. The topics covered ranged from reviews about student teaching and learning, to curricular research, to research on mentoring. Seven of the reviews were about the extant research on specialty education in nursing.

Table 1.4 Nursing Care Delivery

Title	*Author(s)*	*Volume & Pages*
Nursing Staff Turnover, Stress, and Satisfaction: Models, Measures, and Management	Hinshaw, A. S., & Atwood, J. R.	*1*, 133–153
Interorganizational Relations Research in Nursing Care Delivery Systems	Krueger, J. C.	*1*, 155–180
Assessment of Quality of Nursing Care	Lang, N. M., & Clinton, J. F.	*2*, 135–163
Evaluation of Primary Nursing	Giovannetti, P.	*4*, 127–151
Nurse Practitioners and Primary Care Research: Promises and Pitfalls	Shamansky, S. L.	*3*, 107–125
Nursing Administration Research, Part One: Pluralities of Persons	Schultz, P. R., & Miller, K. L.	*8*, 133–158
Information Processing in Nursing Practice	Grier, M. R.	*2*, 265–287
Public Health Nursing Evaluation, Education, and Professional Issues, 1977–1981	Highriter, M. E.	*2*, 165–189
Critical Care Nursing	Dracup, K.	*5*, 107–133
Home Health Care	Barkauskas, V. H.	*8*, 103–132
Nurse Anesthesia Care	Catchpole, M.	*9*, 135–155
Nursing Centers	Riesch, S. K.	*10*, 145–162
Nursing Research and the Study of Health Policy	Milio, N. R.	*2*, 291–306
Acquired Immunodeficiency Syndrome	Turner, J. G.	*8*, 195–210
Cost-Effectiveness Analysis in Nursing Research	Fagin, C. M., & Jacobsen, B. S.	*3*, 215–238
Variable Costs of Nursing Care in Hospitals	Sovie, M. D.	*6*, 131–150

Table 1.5 Professional Issues in Nursing

Title	*Author(s)*	*Volume & Pages*
Socialization and Roles in Nursing	Conway, M. E.	*1*, 183–208
The Staff Nurse Role	Chaska, N.	*10*, 185–203
Leadership in Nursing	McCloskey, J. C., & Molen, M. T.	*5*, 177–202
Men in Nursing	Christman, L. P.	*6*, 193–205
Faculty Practice	Chickadonz, G. H.	*5*, 137–151
Acquired Immunodeficiency Syndrome	Turner, J. G.	*8*, 195–210
Drug and Alcohol Abuse in Nurses	Sullivan, E. J., & Handley, S. M.	*10*, 113–125

Table 1.6 Nursing Education, Continuing Education, and Faculty

Title	*Author(s)*	*Volume & Pages*
Research on the Teaching–Learning Process in Nursing Education	de Tornyay, R.	*2*, 193–210
Research on Nursing Students	Schwirian, P. M.	*2*, 211–237
Curricular Research in Nursing	Stember, M. L.	*2*, 239–262
Research on Continuing Education in Nursing	Kuramoto, A. L.	*3*, 149–170
Doctoral Education of Nurses: Historical Development, Programs, and Graduates	Murphy, J. M.	*3*, 171–189
Nontraditional Nursing Education	Lenburg, C. B.	*4*, 195–215
Computer-Aided Instruction in Nursing Education	Chang, B. L.	*4*, 217–233
Teaching Clinical Judgment	Tanner, C. A.	*5*, 153–173
Mentorship	Vance, C., & Olson, R.	*9*, 175–200
Psychiatric-Mental Health Nursing Education	Loomis, M. E.	*6*, 153–166
Community Health Nursing Education	Flynn, B. C.	*6*, 167–190
Parent–Child Nursing Education	Alexander, C.	*7*, 157–170
Education for Critical Care Nursing	Kinney, M. R.	*8*, 161–176
Occupational Health Nursing Education	Rogers, B.	*9*, 159–171
Nursing Research Education	Jamann-Riley, J. S.	*8*, 177–191
Nursing Administration Education	Anderson, R. A.	*10*, 165–181
Faculty Productivity	Andreoli, K. G., & Musser, L. A.	*4*, 177–193

International Nursing Research

During the first decade of the *ARNR* series, five reviews of studies done outside the United States were published (see Table 1.7). Two of these were general reviews about international nursing research and the others critiqued the work done in Scotland, Canada, and the Philippines.

CONTEXTUAL CHANGES IN NURSING RESEARCH: 1982–1992

Many changes have occurred in the field of nursing over the past decade. During the next 10 years of the *ARNR*, some of these positive changes in nursing should be reflected as substantive changes in the quality of the studies that are reviewed for this series. When the first volume of the *ARNR* went to press in 1982, there were 22 doctoral programs in nursing (Murphy, 1985). The total number of nurses with earned doctoral degrees was only about 3,650 (ANA, 1984). Many of these nurses did not develop programs of research with attendant regular and systematic output of research publications. In fact, the more common approach was to do the dissertation research and perhaps none or one subsequent study during the career. The major federal source for research funding was the Division of Nursing in the Health Resources & Services Administration. The annual funding levels for public support of nursing research ranged between $5 and $8 million per year. During 1984 to 1986, a massive effort by organized nursing led to the creation of the National Center for Nursing Research (NCNR) in April 1986. This event catapulted nursing research into a new era of development and national prestige (Stevenson, 1988) that has had significant impact on every component of the discipline. It is probably more accurate to see the opening of the NCNR as the

Table 1.7 International Nursing Research

Title	*Author(s)*	*Volume & Pages*
Nursing Research in Scotland: A Critical Review	Hockey, L., & Clark, M. O.	*2,* 307–324
Nursing Education Research in Canada	Allemang, M. M., & Cahoon, M. C.	*4,* 261–278
Nursing Research in the Philippines	Williams, P. D.	*6,* 263–291
International Nursing Research	Meleis, A. I.	*5,* 205–227
International Nursing Research	Henry, B. M., & Nagelkerk, J. M.	*10,* 207–230

concrete symbol of the new era rather than the cause or the effect of the new era. In fact, many events, activities, and products of earlier efforts came to fruition in the mid-1980s. Evidence of growth and change includes: the NCNR grant budget for 1992 was $40 million (compared to $8 million in 1986) and the National Research Service Award (NRSA) budget was $4.4 million. In contrast to the 22 doctoral programs of 1981–1982 (Murphy, 1985), there were 53 doctoral programs in nursing in late 1991 (Bednash, Berlin, & Haux, 1991). The estimated number of doctoral students in nursing enrolled during 1990 was 2,683 (Bednash et al., 1991). Note that the number of students enrolled in doctoral programs in 1990 more than equaled the 1985 figure for the entire population of nurses with an earned doctorate. The estimated number of nurses with an earned doctorate in 1988 was 6,416 (Division of Nursing, 1990). Postdoctoral opportunities have increased and so has the number of nurses making use of these opportunities. The postdoctoral opportunities afforded by the Robert Wood Johnson Foundation clinical scholars program and postdoctoral individual and institutional NRSAs have enhanced the research expertise of nurse investigators. In the early years of the 1990s many more nurses appear to be committed to a sustained program of research.

Other changes occurred between 1982 and 1992. The original two regional research societies in the West and Midwest flourished. New nursing research societies were formed in the South and along the Eastern seaboard (Stevenson, 1987) and they are growing rapidly. New research journals have been published and nearly all nursing journals feature selected research reports. Myriad nursing research conferences each year provide a stepping stone to the development of manuscripts for submission to various journals. The promotion and tenure criteria in all of higher education has provided an impetus for development and maintenance of programs of research by nurses in academe. Many large health care agencies have nursing research offices or departments and employ qualified research staff to guide clinical studies. Small grant programs, such as those supported by the American Nurses Foundation and Sigma Theta Tau International, together with the NRSA mechanism, have provided funding to doctoral students and persons with new doctorates to do early projects that will launch their programs of research.

One outcome of this significant increase in the cadre of career nurse-researchers and the heightened level of their research activity should be a greater demand for and use of comprehensive critical reviews in many topic areas. During the second decade, Werley's dream and Springer's risk should come to yield even greater benefits. The ARNR series should enjoy an ever-growing role in knowledge development by improving the efficiency with which investigators conduct their literature reviews and by providing the community of nursing scholars with recommendations of experts about promising areas for future research.

FROM THE 10th ANNIVERSARY INTO THE NEXT DECADE

In its initial 10 years, the *Annual Review of Nursing Research* has been a synthesis, critique, and celebration of the output of research by nurses. The sense of pride in development of knowledge by nurses and the need to show the world that nurses do produce research were powerful motivators throughout the 1980s. As nursing research has evolved and matured, the more pressing need now would seem to be for comprehensive review and synthesis of specifically focused segments of literature that will have a significant impact on knowledge development for nursing.

Nursing (practice) research is directed to answering questions about health promotion, disease prevention, and risk reduction of persons in all age groups. It is directed toward answering questions about care, prevention of iatrogenesis, relief of symptoms, and improvement in quality of life of persons with health deficits. It is directed toward answering questions about optimizing the growth, development, and quality of survival of all ages from low-birth-weight and drug-damaged newborns to the frail elderly (National Center for Nursing Research, 1990). It is different from and complementary to the research agendas in medical research (National Institutes of Health [NIH] Task Force on Nursing Research, 1984; 1989). It is concerned, not only with the individual patient, but with the family, the environment, and the community as these relate to health.

The scientific discipline of nursing has gone through myriad growing pains over the past decade. Most of the outcomes are positive, as indicated in the earlier discussion about the environmental context of nursing knowledge development during the 1980s. The future should hold much promise for more and better research, which, in turn, should lead to increasingly comprehensive reviews focused on narrower topics. More highly educated investigators will conduct more theoretically connected and rigorously crafted studies. Furthermore, these investigators will be involved in programs of research such that a series of studies will build upon one another. If these predictions come true, the integrative critical reviews should be even more valuable than heretofore. Comprehensive reviews of research should lead to more research utilization in the practice arena, in nursing care delivery, in nursing education, and in the public policy arena.

ACKNOWLEDGMENTS

The author wishes to express appreciation to Drs. Harriet H. Werley and Joyce J. Fitzpatrick for their help in putting together the historical aspects of this chapter and for reviewing an early draft of the manuscript. Acknowledgment is also given to Misi Mitchell for her dedicated technical assistance.

REFERENCES

American Nurses' Association. (1981). *Nurses with doctorates*. Final report of Grant No. (5 Rol NU00661), Division of Nursing, U.S. Department of Health and Human Services. Kansas City, MO: Author.

American Nurses' Association. (1984). *Directory of nurses with doctoral degrees*. Kansas City, MO: Author.

Bednash, G. B., Berlin, L. E., & Haux, S. C. (1991). *Institutional Data Systems: 1990–1991 Enrollment and Graduations in Baccalaureate and Graduate Programs in Nursing*. Washington, DC: American Association of Colleges of Nursing.

Division of Nursing, Bureau of Health Professions. (1990). *The Registered Nurse Population: 1988*. U.S. Department of Health and Human Services, Public Health Service. Rockville, MD: Author.

Cooper, H. M. (1982). Scientific guidelines for conducting integrative research reviews. *Review of Educational Research, 52,* 291–302.

Eisdorfer, C. (Ed.) (1980). *Annual Review of Gerontology and Geriatrics*. New York, NY: Springer Publishing Co.

Ellis, R. (1984). Philosophic inquiry. In H. H. Werley & J. J. Fitzpatrick (Eds.), *Annual Review of Nursing Research Vol. 1*. (pp. 211–228). New York, NY: Springer Publishing Co.

Fitzpatrick, J. J., & Taunton, R. L. (Eds.). (1987). *Annual Review of Nursing Research*. (Vol. 5). New York, NY: Springer Publishing Co.

Fitzpatrick, J. J., Taunton, R. L., & Benoliel, J. Q. (Eds.). (1988). *Annual Review of Nursing Research*. (Vol. 6). New York, NY: Springer Publishing Co.

Fitzpatrick, J. J., Taunton, R. L., & Benoliel, J. Q. (Eds.). (1989). *Annual Review of Nursing Research*. (Vol. 7). New York, NY: Springer Publishing Co.

Fitzpatrick, J. J., Taunton, R. L., & Benoliel, J. Q. (Eds.). (1990). *Annual Review of Nursing Research*. (Vol. 8). New York, NY: Springer Publishing Co.

Fitzpatrick, J. J., Taunton, R. L., & Benoliel, J. Q., & Jacox, A. K. (Eds.). (1991). *Annual Review of Nursing Research*. (Vol. 9). New York, NY: Springer Publishing Co.

Fitzpatrick, J. J., Taunton, R. L., & Jacox, A. K. (Eds.). (1992). *Annual Review of Nursing Research*. (Vol. 10). New York, NY: Springer Publishing Co.

Murphy, J. F. (1985). In H. H. Werley & J. J. Fitzpatrick (Eds.) *Annual Review of Nursing Research (Vol. 3)*. (pp. 171–189). New York, NY: Springer Publishing Co.

National Center for Nursing Research. (April 13, 1990). *Mission*. Bethesda, MD: Author.

National Institutes of Health. (1984). *Task Force on Nursing Research: Report to the Director 1984*. Bethesda, MD: Author.

National Institutes of Health. (1989). *Report of the 1989 NIH Task Force on Nursing Research*. NIH Publication #89-487. Bethesda, MD: Author.

Stevenson, J. S. (1987). Forging a research discipline. *Nursing Research, 36,* 60–63.
Stevenson, J. S. (1988). Knowledge development in nursing: Into era II. *Journal of Professional Nursing, 3*(3), 152–162.
Werley, H. H. & Fitzpatrick, J. J. (Eds.). (1984). *Annual Review of Nursing Research.* New York, NY: Springer Publishing Co.
Werley, H. H., & Fitzpatrick, J. J. (Eds). (1985). *Annual Review of Nursing Research.* New York, NY: Springer Publishing Co.
Werley, H. H., Fitzpatrick, J. J., & Taunton, R. L. (Eds). (1986). *Annual Review of Nursing Research.* New York, NY: Springer Publishing Co.

PART I

Research on Nursing Practice

Chapter 2

Urinary Incontinence in Older Adults

KATHLEEN A. MCCORMICK
OFFICE OF THE FORUM FOR QUALITY
AND EFFECTIVENESS IN HEALTH CARE
AGENCY FOR HEALTH CARE POLICY AND RESEARCH

MARY H. PALMER
NATIONAL INSTITUTES OF HEALTH
NATIONAL INSTITUTE ON AGING

CONTENTS

It is estimated that approximately 10 million Americans are incontinent of urine, and the costs of managing incontinence are about $10 billion annually (Hu, 1990). Although the exact mechanism of the development of urinary incontinence is not completely understood, several types of incontinence have been identified. The International Continence Society established a standardized definition for urinary incontinence: ". . . a condition in which involuntary loss of urine is a social or hygienic problem and is objectively demonstrable" (International Continence Society, 1988, p. 17). Additionally, four types of urinary incontinence were defined by the International Continence Society. These include stress incontinence, "involuntary loss of urine occurring when, in the absence of a detrusor contraction, the intravesical pressure exceeds the maximum urethral pressure"; urge incontinence, "involuntary loss of urine associated with a strong urge to void"; overflow incontinence, "involuntary loss of urine associated with over distension of the bladder"; and reflex incontinence, "loss of urine due to detrusor hyperreflexia and/or involuntary urethral relaxation in the absence of the sensation usually associated with the desire to micturate" (International Continence Society, 1988, p. 17). Another type of incontinence described in the literature, especially with elderly, institutionalized populations, is functional incontinence. It is defined as "urinary leakage associated with inability (because of impairment of cognitive or physical functioning), psychological unwillingness, or environmental barriers to toilets" (Ouslander, 1989, p. 252).

Age alone does not cause incontinence. However, proportionally more older adults are incontinent than younger adults (National Institutes of Health Consensus Development Conference, 1990). The natural history and development of incontinence is not understood, although it is associated with increasing functional impairment (Mohide, 1986) and is an indicator of disability (Jagger, Clarke, & Davies, 1986). Not surprising, the prevalence of urinary incontinence is estimated to be 50% in the long-term care setting, where the majority of residents have a functional or cognitive impairment (Kane, Ouslander, & Abrass, 1989). In contrast, it is reported to be present in 9% of the community-dwelling population (Harris, 1986).

Traditionally, nurses have been the health care professionals primarily responsible for the management and care of incontinent adults in institutional and community settings. Because of widely held assumptions that incontinence is caused by old age and is not reversible, the goal of many nursing strategies has been to keep the person clean and dry. Even among affected individuals a sense of futility tends to prevail (Mitteness, 1987a). Many incontinent older adults do not seek medical help and rely on self-management strategies (Herzog & Fultz, 1988). Understanding the cognitive organization of incontinence by community-dwelling older adults is essential in treatment options for incontinence. Mitteness (1987b) found that elaborate plans are made to avoid detection by peers and others while little effort is made to seek medical help.

It was not until the 1980s in the United States that nurse researchers systematically began to investigate the phenomenon of urinary incontinence in older adults. Major areas of research have been assessment methodologies and treatment modalities as well as the financial and psychologic effects of incontinence on health care providers, the affected adults, and family members.

The focus of this chapter is to critically review salient research on urinary incontinence in adults residing in two settings: community and long-term care. Research on the incidence and prevalence of incontinence, assessment, and treatment involving self-management and staff-management strategies of urinary incontinence has been included. Also, nursing research concerning management strategies used solely to contain incontinence, such as appliances and equipment, is discussed.

Several sources were used to identify the relevant studies. The National Library of Medicine's bibliography compiled for the National Consensus Conference on Incontinence in Adults listed 707 journal articles and monographs, from 1983 to 1988, using the key words: urinary incontinence, aged, middle-age, adult. A MEDLINE computerized search was done, from 1985 to 1990, using key words: incontinence, urinary, adults, nursing, dysfunction. From 1985 to 1990, an AGELINE, which is the computerized database of the American Association of Retired Persons, also was executed. A manual search of the International Nursing Index, from 1983 to 1990, yielded no additional citations, using the key words: elimination, urinary alterations, and potential for.

INCIDENCE AND PREVALENCE OF URINARY INCONTINENCE

Little nursing research regarding the incidence and prevalence of urinary incontinence has been reported. Wells and Diokno (1989) noted that no incidence data exist to determine whether urinary incontinence is a unique late-life phenomenon or a process of dysfunctional voiding throughout the life span. Also, little is known about the process of spontaneous remission of incontinence, although it has been reported in one community study. Herzog, Diokno, Brown, Normolle, and Brock (1990) found a 12% remission rate for community-dwelling women and a 30% rate for men.

In one study regarding the prevalence of incontinence in healthy, perimenopausal women (N = 232), 34% (n = 78) reported at least monthly incontinence; the most common type was stress incontinence (Burgio, Matthews, & Engel, 1988). There also are reports of the prevalence of urinary incontinence in community-dwelling, older adults. However, findings often cannot be generalized or compared owing to differences in methods and definitions used for incontinence. For example, in the National Health Interview Survey, 5,637 interviews with adults over the age of 65 years were conducted regarding urinary problems (Harris, 1986). The questions were directed at obtaining information regarding the control of urinary elimination and frequency of any difficulty in control. Herzog et al. (1990) were interested in determining the type and severity of incontinence in noninstitutionalized older adults. They reported the results of one segment of the Medical, Epidemiologic, and Social Aspects of Aging (MESA) Project in which the prevalence of self-reported incontinence in 1,956 subjects was 37.7% in females and 18.9% in males. Males (35.2%) had a higher prevalence of uninhibited bladder contractions than females (7.9%), although incontinent females (12.2%) had a higher prevalence of uninhibited bladder contractions than continent females (4.9%) (Diokno, Brown, Brock, Herzog, & Normolle, 1988).

The voiding patterns in males were investigated in the United Kingdom (Sommer et al., 1990). Five hundred seventy-two men between the ages of 20 and 79 years received a mailed questionnaire about obstructive and irritative urologic symptoms, including urge incontinence. Of the 337 males who completed the questionnaire, 35 men reported urge incontinence (10%) with the prevalence increasing with age; 20% of the males in their 70s had self-reported urge incontinence. Interestingly, none of the subjects sought medical help for treatment or relief from the incontinence.

As Mohide (1986) noted in a discussion of the prevalence of incontinence, varying levels of prevalence may reflect the differences in questions used regarding any incontinence versus severe incontinence, the inclusion or exclusion of external catheter use in the definition, and the source from which information is obtained (i.e., medical records, self-reports of subjects, health care professionals).

ASSESSMENT OF INCONTINENCE

Urinary incontinence is not considered a disease entity; rather it is a condition or symptom (Bates et al., 1979). Assessment studies have focused not only on incontinence itself but on the antecedents of incontinence (factors preceding incontinence) as well as the consequences of the phenomenon.

Antecedents of Incontinence

Wells, Brink, and Diokno (1987) found that stress incontinence was the most prevalent type of incontinence in 200 community-dwelling women, aged 55 years and over, who self-reported being incontinent of urine. The women reported antecedent events of increased abdominal pressure with a cough, changing position, and so forth. Also, stress incontinence was confirmed on physical examination with leakage of urine during a cough test in the supine and standing positions. Before treatment protocols were instituted, diagnoses were formed according to clinical criteria. A combination of urge and stress incontinence was present in 27% of the sample. Pure stress incontinence was present in 66% of the sample; over a third of the sample had atrophic vaginitis.

Weakness of the pelvic muscle has been implicated in the occurrence of urine loss. To determine the strength of the pelvic floor muscle, a digital test has been developed (Brink, Sampselle, Wells, Diokno, & Gillis, 1989) to rate the strength of the contraction on a scale of 0 (no contraction) to 4 (strong contraction). Test–retest reliability for 338 noninstitutionalized women between the ages of 55 and 90 years with complaints of urinary incontinence was $r = 0.65$, $p < 0.01$. Interrater reliability was $r = 0.90$, $p < 0.01$.

The digital rating scale is similar to a previously developed scale designed to measure the strength and duration of contraction of the pelvic muscle, the tone of the muscle during the contraction, and position of the examiner's finger during the examination (Worth, Dougherty, & McKey, 1986). This scale was used with young women between the ages of 18 and 37 years who attended a family planning clinic. These scales are attempts by nurses to standardize and objectively measure pelvic muscle strength during clinical examination.

A device, the intravaginal balloon device (IVBD), was developed to objectively measure the strength of the pelvic muscle (Dougherty, Abrams, & McKey, 1986). The strength of the pelvic muscle did not decrease with age in a sample of 20 volunteers between the ages of 22 and 58 years. The women were recruited from the community and had a negative history for use of hormones and surgical repairs to pelvic structures. Further testing of this device with older women and women who report stress incontinence is needed.

Intact neurologic control of micturition is considered an essential component to continence (Wein, 1986). Neurologic impairment has been associated with the development of urinary incontinence (Ouslander, 1989).

Molander and colleagues (1989) attempted to determine the degree of neurologic impairment in community-dwelling women with urinary incontinence. A random sample of 6,000 women from the birth cohorts 1900 to 1920, living in Goteburg, Sweden, were surveyed regarding urinary incontinence and other related symptoms. Of 4,206 women, 16.9% of the first 150 who reported incontinence on a questionnaire were invited to have neurologic and urodynamic evaluation of their incontinence. An age-matched comparison group of continent women underwent the same examinations. There were no differences in neuropathologic findings between the two groups. The authors concluded that neurologic dysfunction was an uncommon cause of incontinence in the community. This finding supports the Brocklehurst, Andrews, Richards, and Laycock (1985) conclusion that incontinence in adult subjects ($N = 13.5$) following postcerebral vascular accident was due to mobility-impairment and dependency on others rather than to impairments in neurologic functioning.

Measures of Severity of Incontinence

Outpatient. There is no consensus in the literature on measurement of the severity of incontinence. There have been attempts, however, to quantify the amount of urine loss and to monitor the frequency of incontinent episodes. Parkin and Davis (1986) developed a visual analogue scale with values ranging from 0 to 100. Women ($N = 35$) were asked to indicate the severity of their incontinence on this scale before urodynamic examination. There were significant differences between two groups of women. The women with urge incontinence perceived a higher severity to their incontinence than did women with stress incontinence. Frazer, Sutherst, and Holland (1987) used a visual analogue scale ranging from 0 to 100 to measure the severity of incontinence with 110 women prior to urodynamic testing. No distinct differences were found in the rating of severity of incontinence between women with urge incontinence and women with stress incontinence. Women with urge incontinence had a higher degree of wetness than did women with stress incontinence, as measured by a perineal pad-weighing test. The researchers concluded that subjective factors may play a role in the perception of the symptoms of incontinence. Frazer, Haylen, and Sutherst (1989) attempted to determine the relationship between the subjective assessment of the amount of urine loss using an analogue scale and an objective measurement of urine loss through a 2-hour perineal, pad-weighing procedure. They found no relationship between the women's perception of severity of urine loss and objective measurement of urine loss over a 2-hour testing period. The authors recommended that objective measures be used to obtain accurate information in the assessment of incontinence. Clearly, more research is needed to determine the usefulness of a visual analogue scale in the assessment of incontinence.

Quantification of urine loss has been a perplexing problem for clinicians in assessing incontinence. There are reports in the literature of the discrepancy between self-report of fluid loss and quantified measures of urine loss. Fantl, Harkins, Wyman, Choi, and Taylor (1987) described a perineal pad weighing method to quantify urine loss. Sixty-seven noninstitutionalized ambulatory women who were referred to a continence clinic participated in the study. Each woman was first instructed to empty her bladder, a straight catheter was passed to remove residual urine, and subsequently the bladder was filled to capacity with room-temperature normal saline. Perineal pads were secured and the woman was instructed to perform a series of exercises and maneuvers. The pads were measured at the end of the test. Women with sphincter incompetence tended to lose smaller amounts of urine than women who experienced bladder contractions that emptied the bladder partially or completely. The authors noted that within-patient variability was a limitation of the study. Bladder-filling volumes differed statistically between test–retest within diagnostic groups. The authors suggested that factors beyond their control such as volitional control of continence, patient cooperation during provocative maneuvers, and physiologic factors of sphincter fatigue could explain this finding.

Ekelund, Bergstrom, Milsom, Norlen, and Rignell (1988) studied the ability of 34 older women (average age 79 years) to perform a 48-hour, perineal pad test at home. The women were instructed to record the time and weight of the pad at each changing. They were also instructed to record their activity level and degree of incontinence. To evaluate the reliability of weighing, 15 women were instructed to seal their pads in watertight bags and return them to the clinic for repeat weighing. The correlation between the two weights was high, $r = 0.99$. The authors noted that certain deficits such as poor vision and cognitive impairments would act as a barrier to this assessment technique for incontinence in community-dwelling older adults.

Wyman, Choi, Harkins, Wilson, and Fantl (1988) described a self-monitoring technique to assess the frequency of continent and incontinent voidings. Women between the ages of 55 and 86 years who were participating in a behavioral management clinical trial for urinary incontinence were given a urinary diary to record voiding behavior for 2 weeks prior to urodynamic testing. The findings indicated that the specific voiding behaviors such as diurnal frequency, nocturnal micturition frequency, and number of incontinent episodes were reproducible from week to week. However, women who had unstable bladders, that is, women who experienced uninhibited bladder contractions, were less consistent in recording the number of urinary leakages than were women with sphincter incompetence. Women also had difficulty in recording very slight amounts of urine loss because they were unsure whether to document very slight incontinent voiding. These data confirm that consistent definitions of incontinence are essential to achieve meaningful information.

In contrast to the high prevalence of incompetent sphincters among women with complaints of incontinence, males exhibit a higher prevalence of urge incontinence, as noted in the previously mentioned MESA study (Diokno et al., 1988). During cystometric testing, uninhibited bladder contractions were evident in 35% of the males as compared to 7.9% of the females. Another interesting finding was that the level of postvoid, residual urine volume was not associated with continence status. Thus, varying levels of postvoid, residual urine were present in continent as well as incontinent subjects. The findings may reflect the effect of self-management strategies, such as fluid restriction, which are employed by the community-dwelling, older adult.

Long-Term Care. The predominant type of incontinence appears to be different in the nursing home population when compared to the community setting. Resnick, Yalla, and Laurino (1989) found that detrusor hyperreflexia is the most common physical sign of incontinence in this setting. They also delineated two subsets of this dysfunction: one in which the detrusor contractility is intact and the other in which contractility is impaired (DHIC).

Mental impairment in nursing home residents creates difficulty in obtaining information in assessing incontinence; thus, the reliance on documentation of staff becomes necessary (Miller, 1990). Documentation of incontinence in the medical record can be inconsistent (Palmer, McCormick, & Langford, 1989; Petrucci, McCormick, & Scheve, 1987) or nonexistent (Pannill, Williams, & Davis, 1988). Objective and reliable monitoring of incontinence is as necessary in the assessment and treatment of affected adults in the institutionalized setting as it is in the outpatient setting.

The use of bladder charts is a method to obtain information regarding the time of an incontinent episode, the amount of fluid loss, and other information such as the adult's awareness of the incident. Ouslander, Urman, and Uman (1986) described the Incontinence Monitoring Record (IMR), which allowed quick documentation of incontinent episodes. It was designed for ease of use by the primary caregiver in the nursing home (geriatric nursing assistant). Miller (1990) tested the interrater reliability of the Incontinence Monitoring Record in a 129-bed nursing home with 32 nursing assistants. Interrater reliability was high: 89% on 55 checks over a 24-hour period. The authors recommended including an additional column entitled, "Unsuccessful Attempts to Void," to enhance sensitivity of the tool.

O'Donnell, Beck, and Walls (1990) reported another noninvasive assessment technique of incontinence. An electronic incontinence sensor was placed in an absorbent pad worn by the patient and the sensor transmitter was positioned for the convenience of the patient. The frequency of incontinence and volume of urine loss were measured continuously for 10 days. Significantly more incontinent episodes occurred during the evening shift when compared to the day and night shifts; however, the largest fluid volume losses occurred on the night shift. There was 99.7% accuracy in detecting wetness when compared to hourly wet checks. The authors noted that most treatment options that feature scheduled toileting, regardless of fixed or flexible schedule, occurred predominantly during the day shift, when incontinent episodes are occurring at their lowest rate. They suggested coordination of treatment schedule with the individual voiding patterns for effective treatment and reduction in wetness episodes. The findings indicated a need to explore the effectiveness of intervention studies conducted during the evening and night hours.

Algorithms for assessing incontinence have been developed primarily for use by physicians (Hilton, 1987; Hilton & Stanton, 1981; Ouslander, 1986). Ouslander (1986) described an algorithm developed to assess incontinence in males and females that could be used by a nurse practitioner in a long-term care setting. This algorithm was particularly designed to be practical and cost-effective in the identification of: (a) reversible causes of incontinence; (b) those who required more extensive evaluation; and (c) treatment that did not require formal urodynamic testing. The algorithm was designed to include the use of bedside invasive diagnostic tests such as postvoid, residual, urine volume, and bladder filling to determine capacity and leakage under stress maneuvers. Ouslander reported that a nurse practitioner successfully treated 86% of 120 patients using the algorithm.

The presence of 100 cc in the bladder after voiding has been considered indicative of obstruction or a hypotonic bladder (Wyman, 1988). However, Starer and Libow (1988) found that a postvoid, residual volume of 100 cc or greater did not predict the type of bladder dysfunction. They also found that many of the subjects had a difficult time emptying their bladders prior to the evaluation; therefore, a concern regarding the accuracy of assessment of the bladder-emptying ability was raised. This finding supports Diokno's (1990) contention that there is no established amount of residual urine volume that is significant in the diagnosis of urinary incontinence.

Consequences of Urinary Incontinence

Outpatient. The psychologic effects of incontinence have been of interest to researchers in the United Kingdom and the United States. It should be noted that the majority of findings are from studies where the samples are drawn from individuals who sought help for incontinence. The majority of incontinent individuals, however, do not seek help; therefore, the ability to generalize from the findings is limited. Wyman, Harkins, and Fantl (1990) noted that: (a) standardized measurement tools have not been refined; (b) age, gender, and ethnic differences in perceived impact should be investigated; (c) differences in impact between those who seek help and those who do not should be explored; (d) the influence of comorbidity on the psychologic impact of incontinence should be explored; (e) the relationship of perceived impact and different types of incontinence should be investigated; and (f) effect of treatment on the psychologic impact of urinary incontinence should be determined.

In 1982 Norton reported that community-dwelling women ($N = 55$) who attended a continence clinic felt that incontinence affected at least one sphere of their lives: physical health, mental well-being, ability to cope with domestic chores, social life, relationship with the family, intimate relations, work, the way one dresses, and restriction of activities. The women reported more effects to mental well-being than to physical well-being. Also, they reported that they restricted activities out of fear of an incontinent episode. The severity of urine loss was not associated with the magnitude of the physiologic effects. Norton noted that individual responses were varied and could not predict the effect of incontinence on individual subjects. These findings support those of Harris (1986): incontinent, older adults were likely to participate less frequently in social and church activities outside the home.

Wyman, Harkins, Choi, Taylor, and Fantl (1987) measured the psychologic impact of incontinence on 69 noninstitutionalized women who participated in a clinical trial on incontinence. The measurement tool used was a 26-item Incontinence Impact Questionnaire (Wyman et al., 1987) that clustered items into three broad categories: activities of daily living, social interactions, and self-perceptions. Self-perceptions and activities were most affected by incontinence. Many women felt a moderate to severe impact of incontinence on their mental health, and they restricted activities in unfamiliar places. There were significant correlations between the scores on the questionnaire and frequency of incontinent episodes and quantification of fluid loss. The authors cautioned, however, that the relationship was modest and psychologic impact was not directly proportional to the objective measures of severity of incontinence, such as quantification of fluid loss.

Males were included in the MESA study of the relationship between urinary incontinence and psychologic distress (Herzog et al., 1988). It was found that continent women had the highest psychologic well-being and life satisfaction. Women with more severe incontinence, as measured by the number of days incontinent and the amount of fluid loss with each episode, had more psychologic distress. Incontinent males also experienced more psychologic distress than continent males, but the relationship did not hold with increasing severity. The authors attributed the lack of significant findings to the small sample size of moderately and severely incontinent males. The authors further cautioned that women who reported incontinence and psychologic distress also tended to be more physically impaired than continent women. Further research on the relationship of psychologic and personality factors to reports of incontinence severity needs to be conducted.

Long-Term Care. Yu (1987) developed a tool, The Incontinence Stress Index, to measure the psychologic impact of incontinence in women. The Incontinence Stress Index consisted of four factors: agitated depressive symptoms, retarded depressive symptoms, feelings of abandonment, and somatic concerns and activities related to urinary incontinence. The scale was pilot-tested with 30 females residing in long-term care facilities. It was further tested with 96 female residents of long-term care facilities (Yu, Kaltreider, Hu, Igou, & Craighead, 1989). It was refined to 20 items with three factors: depressive, aesthetic/somatic, and social. Severely cognitively impaired women were unable to complete the questionnaire, but cognitively intact women reported that they felt stress from being incontinent and that staff and other patients avoided them. This scale requires testing with larger samples of cognitively intact incontinent adults in various settings. Also, albeit a challenging endeavor, a measure of stress should be developed for cognitively impaired incontinent elderly.

TREATMENTS FOR INCONTINENCE

Outpatient Setting

About half of the incontinent, older adults in the community do not seek medical help to treat or manage incontinence (National Institutes of Health Consensus Development Conference, 1990). Mitteness (1987b) reported that older adults attempt to hide their incontinence by remaining outside the medical system, keeping a distance from others through social isolation, and using cognitive maps of public toilets when they venture out. Strategies to encourage incontinent adults to seek help are needed as well as adequate resources within the community to provide information about incontinence and appropriate referral and evaluation.

Nursing/behavioral treatments currently available to change the continence outcomes of community-dwelling adults are categorized into four major interventions: (a) habit training, (b) bladder retraining, and (c) biofeedback.

Habit Training. Habit training, also called scheduled voiding or temporal voiding, involves a fixed schedule, usually every 2 to 4 hours, for bladder emptying (Hadley et al., 1986). Urinary incontinence is avoided by using a fixed schedule to urinate rather than relying on sensations of bladder fullness.

Incontinent, frail, elderly adults in the community have been evaluated and treated with habit training in a geriatric day hospital on a very limited scale (Morishita, 1988). There is a great need to implement well-designed clinical studies investigating the effect of habit training on frequency of incontinence in community-dwelling or home-bound older adults. Prospective studies exploring the effectiveness of habit training on outcomes with larger samples of frail, elderly adults in the community and home care setting are necessary.

Bladder Retraining. Bladder retraining, also known as bladder drill or bladder training, involves a variable schedule of voiding. The individual keeps a bladder record and is encouraged to increase the interval between voidings. Motivation to follow the treatment plan and the ability to understand and interpret body sensations are necessary. This intervention is used to treat urge incontinence (Wells, 1988). The bladder capacity is expected to increase and sensations of urgency are expected to eventually lessen with the expanded voiding intervals.

Castleden, Duffin, Asher, and Yeomenson (1985) studied older adults ($N = 95$) who had unstable detrusor contractions and were placed on a one-half hour or one-hour habit retraining schedule, which was increased by one-half hour after they remained dry for 48 hours. The interval continued to be increased until the subject reached a voiding schedule of 4 hours. Also, they were treated with imipramine, at an initial dose of 25 mg, taken at night and increased during the course of the study. The factors that most affected patient outcome were the mental status and mobility level of the individual. These researchers relied on self-reports of subjects regarding compliance to the schedule and episodes of wetness. Therefore, selection bias (that is, only cognitively intact individuals could comply with the protocol) may have influenced the results. Future research should explore the effects of enhancing mobility and cognitive function on bladder retraining as measured by the level of dryness achieved by the older adults.

Fantl et al. (1991) reported the findings of a randomized clinical trial using bladder training with 123 community-dwelling women. Each woman had a urodynamic assessment. The bladder training consisted of voiding at assigned times, using relaxation and distraction techniques to suppress the urge to void prior to the assigned time. The women were instructed to keep a daily treatment log in which they recorded the number of incontinent episodes. Women with urethral incompetence and women with detrusor instability had a reduction of incontinent episodes by 57%, and the quantity of urine loss was reduced by 54%.

Biofeedback

Biofeedback has been used as a treatment option for stress and urge incontinence and a condition, bladder-sphincter dyssynergia, in which there is lack of synchronization between bladder contraction and urethral sphincter relaxation. Physiologic responses are changed through a process of operant conditioning in which the individual learns by observing the results of the voluntary efforts made to control bladder and sphincter activity (Burgio, Whitehead, & Engel, 1985).

Biofeedback also has been used as treatment for poststroke and postprostatectomy incontinence. Middaugh, Whitehead, Burgio, and Engel (1989) reported that four males, who had a previous stroke and were recruited from the community, successfully maintained continence after participating in biofeedback-assisted bladder retraining. All subjects were able to attain continence by 6 months. Only two subjects were available for a 12-month follow-up and they remained continent. The investigators concluded that the physiologic functioning of the bladder was not changed through training, but the individual was assisted in better management of a low-volume hyperreflexic bladder. Because of the small sample size, the threat of self-selection, lack of control group, and the combined habit training and biofeedback treatment, generalization of the findings are limited. However, the dramatic change in continence status indicates that further investigation of this intervention with a larger sample of males and females is warranted.

Biofeedback was also an effective intervention for 20 males, aged 55 to 87 years, with postprostatectomy incontinence of at least a 6-month duration (Burgio, Stutzman, & Engel, 1989). Eight males had stress incontinence, eight males had urge incontinence, and nine had continuous leakage, and five subjects had a combination of more than one diagnosis. After one or more biofeedback training sessions, there was an average 78% decrease in stress incontinence and an average 80% decrease in urge incontinence. Males with continuous leakage had less successful results. There was an average 17% reduction in leakage for these subjects. The authors suggested that these findings indicated that there was damage to the mechanism of passive control of continence; therefore, candidates for biofeedback should be carefully selected based on the pattern of urine loss over several days. Also, candidates must actively participate in therapy and be motivated to continue the therapy on their own.

Baigis-Smith, Smith, Rose, and Newman (1989) found that biofeedback techniques, habit training, and relaxation techniques provided significant improvement in continence in community-dwelling older adults. A sample of 54 older adults, 45 females and 9 males, who were cognitively intact and motivated to learn pelvic muscle exercises, was recruited to participate in the study through newspaper announcements and presentations at senior centers and nutrition sites.

There were significant decreases in the number of wet episodes after pelvic muscle exercises and biofeedback. There was a statistically significant decrease in the mean number of incontinence episodes. The mean number of incontinence episodes decreased from 17 in baseline to four at the end of treatment. The decreases persisted through a follow-up evaluation at 6 months for 33 subjects available to follow-up. Age was not a significant factor in improvement in this study.

Subject self-selection, lack of randomization, and lack of control group limit the generalizability of these findings. Attrition was a factor in this study, and data were not available on those who dropped out of the study. Therefore, the study results may be biased toward individuals committed to completing the study and complying with the treatment protocol. Also, because the preponderance of subjects were female, sample bias may have affected the results of this study. Because the study included four treatment interventions, it is not possible to determine which intervention provided the improvement in continence.

Burton, Pearce, Burgio, Engel, and Whitehead (1988) reported the findings of a study in which 27 older adult subjects were nonrandomly assigned to one of two interventions by a geriatrician and nurse practitioner after assessment of their incontinence: behavioral training (nurse education) without biofeedback and biofeedback without education. Both groups experienced significant reductions in wetness that were maintained in a 1-month follow-up visit. The reports of reduction in wetness were derived from self-reported bladder records. Self-selection by highly motivated individuals to enroll in a protocol that required multiple visits limits the generalizability of the results. The authors acknowledged that spontaneous improvement was not addressed, although the likelihood of it occurring is slight owing to the long-standing nature of the incontinence and the baseline measure of incontinent episodes. The addition of a control group would help to detect a placebo effect. Replication of the study using objective measures of wetness would provide additional and necessary information regarding the effectiveness of these treatment options.

Treatment therapies vary with types of incontinence, the characteristics and motivation of affected individuals, resources available, and the setting. It continues to be necessary to have experimental, prospective studies with control groups to determine the effectiveness of treatments on outcomes. Also, there is a need to link therapies with economic indicators to determine cost-effectiveness. Further, researchers who measure continence outcomes in community-dwelling subjects need to standardize their method of defining cure, improvement, or percentage improvement in wetness and/or dryness. It is also necessary to realize that outcomes can be described at the end of treatment or at the end of 3-, 6-, or 12-month follow-up.

Long-Term Care Setting

The treatment of incontinence in nursing homes is dependent on the type of incontinence, the characteristics of affected individuals, and availability of the nursing staff (Ouslander, 1990). Cognitive and mobility impairments are highly prevalent among nursing home residents (Ouslander, 1989). The nursing home industry typically is staffed with unskilled workers who have high turnover rates, creating an instability in the quality of care given to the residents (Institute of Medicine, 1986).

Behavioral therapies can be focused on modifying the antecedents or the consequences of incontinence (Burgio & Engel, 1987). Behavioral therapies can differ in the manner in which they are administered (Burgio & Burgio, 1986). Some therapies, such as pelvic muscle exercise, can be self-managed by the individual, and other therapies are staff-managed, especially for cognitively and mobility-impaired individuals. Several behavioral therapies to treat incontinence in adults in the long-term care setting have been developed in recent years, these include: (a) habit training, (b) contingency management, and (c) staff management.

Habit Training. Habit training has been used to treat institutionalized, cognitively impaired adults with functional or urge incontinence (Burgio & Burgio, 1986). The interval between toiletings on this schedule usually is one hour (Hu et al., 1989; Schnelle, Sowell, Hu, & Traughber, 1988). These two randomized, controlled, clinical trials have shown a reduction of one incontinent episode per day. Thus, their findings show that a prompted-voiding program in long-term care is cost-effective.

Habit training may be combined with another form of therapy. Ouslander, Blaustein, Connor, and Pitt (1988) reported findings from a study in which 15 incontinent nursing home residents with a clinical diagnosis of detrusor hyperreflexia were placed on a 6-week trial of habit training combined with medications management. For the first 2 weeks, only habit training was used; for the second 2 weeks, habit training was combined with a placebo; and the final 2 weeks included habit training and administration of a smooth muscle relaxant, oxybutynin. A 2-hour schedule was used: wet episodes decreased significantly with habit training in the first 2 weeks. There was no further significant reduction with the addition of a placebo or drug. The authors noted that the limitations of the study included a small sample size, duration of the study, lack of control over the magnitude and consistency of the treatment, and potentially insensitive outcome measures. This study reflects the complex nature of incontinence in the long-term care setting and identification of factors such as the duration of the study period that may influence outcomes.

Contingency Management. Contingency management, also referred to as behavioral modification, is a consistent and systematic approach of rewarding continent voiding through verbal praise and discouraging incontinence with verbal disapproval (Burgio & Engel, 1987). Contingency management is sometimes combined with the scheduled voiding intervention. Several studies have used prompted-voiding therapy, a form of contingency management with scheduled voiding. This intervention can even be used with cognitively impaired adults.

Many of the protocols for prompted voiding are similar. The subject is approached at a predetermined time and prompted to use the toilet. Assistance to the toilet is provided if necessary and social approval is given for using the toilet. There are differences in procedures, with some protocols using 1-

hour checks (Creason et al., 1989; Hu et al., 1989; Schnelle et al., 1989) and others using 2-hour checks (Engel et al., 1990).

Schnelle et al. (1989) reported that 126 residents of a long-term care facility were assigned to immediate and delayed prompted-voiding therapy groups. The majority of the subjects were cognitively impaired and incapable of independent voiding. Prompted-voiding treatment consisted of hourly checks of the subjects and asking if they were wet or dry. The resident was checked for accuracy and if dry, was given social approval. If the resident was wet, clothing was changed and corrective feedback was given by telling the resident that assistance should have been requested. Residents also were toileted and given additional social reinforcement when they expressed willingness to void. A significant predictor for success of this treatment was the first day's response—low wetness and high appropriate toileting were predictive of high continence outcomes. The authors suggested that residents were not learning new continence skills but responding to increased opportunities in the environment to be continent. They also suggested that nurse managers can use first-day baseline and first-day treatment responses as prognostic criteria to identify residents who would best respond to this therapy. It should be noted that the study population was cognitively impaired; the average score on the Mini-Mental Status Exam (Folstein, Folstein, & McHugh, 1975) was 8.0, on a scale of 0 to 30, where 30 is cognitively intact. This score indicates severe cognitive impairment. Therefore, the amount of responsiveness from such an impaired group to prompting was a promising finding.

Creason et al. (1989) used prompted voiding with a social intervention every waking hour with female nursing home residents. Eighty-five residents (mean age 87 years), who were incontinent of urine for at least 2 weeks, were included in the study. The majority of the sample residents were severely cognitively and functionally impaired. A quasiexperimental design was employed: 30 subjects were assigned to the prompted-voiding and social-reinforcement intervention, 27 subjects were assigned to a socialization group alone, and 28 residents were assigned to a control group. The socialization intervention consisted of 2 to 3 minutes, each hour, of conversing pleasantly with the subject. Prompted-voiding therapy included asking the resident every waking hour if the toilet was needed. A wetness/dryness check was conducted at the same time regardless of the response. The control group also was checked for dryness and continued to receive routine incontinence care, which consisted of checking for incontinence every 2 or 3 hours. Prompted voiding was an effective technique in reducing wet episodes over a 5-week period. The results were similar to those of Schnelle et al. (1989). Immediate response to treatment was not measured in this study as it was with Schnelle et al.; however, after 5 weeks of treatment, significant reduction in incontinence episodes occurred.

Hu et al. (1989) described their protocol as intending to assist subjects in identifying muscular cues of bladder fullness by instructing them to hold their urine until the next check, although they could use a toilet if they notified the research assistant to receive assistance. A randomized, controlled, experimental design investigated the effectiveness of prompted voiding with female residents, aged 65 years and older, at five long-term care facilities. After baseline measures were obtained, 71 females were assigned to a control group and 72 females were assigned to the treatment group. The treatment period lasted 13 weeks and follow-up data were collected at 2, 4, and 6 months posttreatment. There were significant reductions in wet episodes immediately after treatment and throughout the follow-up period. The authors suggested that the treatment group continued to improve because the subjects learned to make self-initiated requests to use the toilet. They found that those who were more severely incontinent improved more than those who were less severely incontinent, and the probability of improvement was greater for subjects with higher Mini-Mental Status Exam scores. Also, subjects who had normal bladder function responded well to training.

Hu et al. (1990) also noted an important finding in that the therapy was labor intensive and there was an increase in labor costs that may have been higher than the savings in laundry costs. This finding supports other research that shows that behavioral therapies are labor intensive and increase costs, at least initially, to the facility (Sowell, Schnelle, Hu, & Traughber, 1987). The balance of costs and benefits of behavioral programs needs to be quantified; however, some benefits such as improved psychologic well-being and increased quality of life from being more continent is difficult to measure. Residents in the Hu et al. (1989) study, benefited from the program with increased dryness and psychologic improvement. The authors suggested that incentives such as financial rewards be given to staff who toilet patients and save money on supplies in order to increase work productivity. Schnelle et al. (1988) noted that medical interventions may augment behavioral therapies, improving the effectiveness of treatment and eventually reducing costs in supplies and labor. Also, the identification of individuals who would benefit from behavioral therapies is necessary for efficient management strategies to be implemented.

Engel et al. (1990) described a 3-year study that augmented a prompted-voiding therapy with several additional procedures. One study analyzed the usefulness of different treatment schedules of prompted voiding on the improvement of incontinence in 41 residents (McCormick, Burgio, Scheve, Hawkins, Leahy, & Engel, in review). Residents who were wet when baseline measures were taken were prompted hourly, and there was a statistically significant improvement over baseline. However, the residents did not maintain this improvement when they were transferred to the home units that used a 2-hour schedule. Residents who were treated with a 2-hour schedule improved and maintained this treatment effect. One group went on to be treated every 3 hours and also continued to improve on this schedule. Residents who were relatively dry while in baseline were prompted on a 3-hour schedule and also significantly improved. This study included a small unmatched sample for treatment schedules and had no controls, and yet the outcomes achieved were the same as the randomized, controlled clinical trials, that is, improvement of one episode per day.

Because many residents in long-term care are cognitively impaired and do not respond to routine prompted-voiding treatment, a study was designed to augment prompted-voiding treatment with a bellpad. A bellpad is an electronic alarm device that rings when wet with urine (McCormick et al., 1992). The results indicated that the bellpad treatment was associated with significantly increased dryness, compared to baseline, in 11 residents. In addition, improved dryness was maintained for up to 3 months in residents remaining on follow-up treatment. These findings indicate that even severely cognitively impaired residents' continence status can be improved with nursing techniques in long-term care. This study should be done with a larger sample and control subjects. The device used in this study also required subjects to be seated most of the day. Other devices that allow more resident mobility should be researched.

Another group in long-term care consists of those who are severely mobility-impaired. They require either two personnel to lift them or the use of a mechanical lift. In a study that monitored the results of prompted-void treatment augmented by a mechanical lift, the costs of incontinence treatment also were documented (McCormick, Cella, Scheve, & Engel, 1990). This study demonstrated that a mechanical lift and a 2-hour toileting schedule improved continence in 10 nursing home residents. Because this incontinence treatment is labor intensive, the cost of treating incontinence increased by $2.90, but the cost of the consequences of incontinence (decubitus ulcers and urinary tract infections) decreased by $13.37 per patient per day. The sample size was small, there was no matched control group, and there was no standard number of treatment days in this study. This study also needs to be expanded.

Staff-management. In the institutional long-term care setting, staff management techniques have been used with success to improve the continence status of elderly residents. Staff management in the institutional setting involves several components (Schnelle, 1991).

Two phases were described in a study to demonstrate the effectiveness of staff management procedures (Burgio et al., 1990). In phase 1, research assistants were taught to administer prompted-voiding treatment. The staff management system included self-monitoring and recording of prompted-voiding activities, supervisory monitoring by the head nurse, and feedback based on group performance and activities. This system was initially effective, but performance began to decline in 4 to 5 months after initiation. In phase 2, another more personalized system was implemented by the same staff to restore staff performance. During phase 2, feedback was provided to each staff member individually. Results showed that once individual feedback was provided, the staff performance exceeded the initial levels achieved in phase 1. In a subsequent study, the monitoring of individual performance was augmented with contingencies. A letter was placed into the nursing staff's personnel file every 3 months praising positive performance and giving disapproval of low performance (Hawkins, Langford, Engel, & Burgio, in review). Results showed that individual feedback plus contingencies produced significant improvements by the number of assigned prompted-voiding checks and toileting episodes completed.

Environmental Modifications

Anecdotal reports abound that in the long-term care setting, environmental modifications to encourage self-toileting behavior, to make toilets accessible, and to develop a positive attitude of the staff improve continence status (Jirovec, Brink, & Wells, 1988; Wells, 1980). However, scant research literature is available to evaluate the accessibility of toilets, the impact of staff attitude, and types of nursing practice on outcomes: this area is worth investigating. Miller (1984, 1985) reported that many nursing practices, which are task-focused, encourage dependency in patients. Miller (1984) postulated that nursing activity was not just a consequence of incontinence (changing patients, removing clothing, etc.), but an antecedent to incontinence ["nursing actions, produces or exacerbates incontinence" (p. 481)]. She also found that patients admitted at the same *level of care* differed in *level of dependency* needs after a month (Miller, 1985, p. 481). Three hospitals were matched by size, admission policy, type of patients, and staffing levels. One hundred sixty-eight patients (M = 80 years old) were evaluated on six nursing units using the CAPES dependency scale. The results indicated that although long-term care patients were similar in dependency needs at admission, those admitted to nursing units where traditional nursing care (i.e., task-oriented care) was practiced were more dependent than their counterparts who were admitted to nursing units where the nursing process and individual care plans were employed. Miller (1985) suggested that dependency is a consequence of traditional nursing practice and can be minimized when individualized plans of care are followed. Miller also found that nursing tasks are designed for the convenience of the staff rather than the good of the patient. This study suggests that restructuring the work in the patient care environment may be indicated, as well as restructuring the system of allocating resources. Miller (1985) noted that in some systems the nursing staff may be penalized for maintaining patient independence by reductions in staffing levels: conversely, the staff is rewarded by caring for highly dependent patients through increases in staff levels. Evaluation studies of patient mix, staffing levels, specific nursing practices, and specific functional outcomes are needed to determine: (a) if incontinence is a nursing-induced iatrogenic condition in long-term care patients; and (b) if incentives exist in current work structures for the nursing staff to provide continence care.

Little is known about the importance of social interaction between the staff and incontinent residents in nursing homes. For example, the effect of social interaction among staff and residents and the prevalence of incontinence has not been studied. Also, the social impact of incontinence on adults in highly structured settings, such as nursing homes and boarding homes, has not been systematically investigated. Concepts such as stigma, motivation to being continent, and importance of personal hygiene have not been the focus of nursing research.

Equipment and Appliances

As mentioned earlier in the discussion of the effectiveness of bellpads and mechanical lifts, equipment can play a vital role in the treatment of incontinence. Not all older adults are appropriate candidates for the behavioral therapies discussed. Many older adults in the long-term care setting are frail or in the terminal stage of a disease, and, therefore, external appliances and indwelling catheters are appropriate. There are few published studies investigating the outcomes with the use of different appliances.

The primary goal of urine-collection devices is to contain urine. A universally accepted external, urine-collection device for women has not been developed, but several designs have been patented (Pieper, Cleland, Johnson, & O'Reilly, 1989).

Ouslander, Greengold, and Chen (1987) reported the findings of a study that investigated the incidence of bacteriuria in institutionalized older males ($N = 97$) who used external catheters to manage incontinence. Four groups were followed prospectively for 6 months: those who wore the catheter continuously ($n = 30$), those who wore the catheter at night ($n = 19$), those who are incontinent and did not use a catheter ($n = 13$), and those who are continent ($n = 30$). The subjects who wore the external catheter continuously had a significantly higher incidence of urinary tract infections than the continent and incontinent who did not wear a catheter. The subjects who wore a catheter at night did not differ significantly from the continent group. The authors found no clinical factors (such as age, functional status, mental status, nutritional status) associated with the development of urinary tract infections. They suggested further research to identify factors that place patients at risk for developing infections. The relationship of the amount and type of fluids ingested orally with the presence of urinary tract infections and incontinence should be explored. The relationship between bacteriuria and incontinence in institutionalized elderly is not clear and should be rigorously explored using a prospective case control design.

Watson (1989) investigated the effectiveness and complications of three urinary sheaths used on six elderly male inpatients over 21 days. No skin breakdown was noted with any of the appliances. There were differences among the sheaths in the average length of time remaining in place. Watson concluded that individual assessment should be performed before a sheath is selected for use. This study should be replicated with a larger sample, other patient outcomes such as the incidence of bacteriuria, and patient acceptance of the appliance.

Indwelling catheter use has been associated with increased incidence of bacteriuria (Warren, 1986). Roe and Brocklehurst (1987) reported on nonphysiologic consequences of the presence of an indwelling catheter. Thirty-six community-dwelling adults were interviewed regarding their knowledge about the catheter's function and location in the body, and the acceptance and consequences of the catheter. They found that the presence of a catheter affected the social life and types of clothes worn by the subjects. The respondents also stated that it took approximately one year to get used to having a catheter. Almost half (42%) said that they were constantly aware of the catheter. The study also revealed that some of the subjects lacked knowledge about proper care of the catheter and potential complications. Provision of essential information regarding the care of the catheter in a systematic manner was suggested by the authors. In a follow-up study, a booklet with information about catheter care was provided to 45 patients (Roe, 1990). There was improvement in knowledge with the provision of the booklet and more emotional coping and adjustment to the catheter.

In people with intractable incontinence, that is, individuals incapable of responding to treatment, one problem is the foul smell associated with incontinence (Norberg, Sandstrom, Norberg, Eriksson, & Sandman, 1984). Reusable and disposable pads and briefs have been developed to contain urine, prevent smell, and improve patient comfort. There have been few studies comparing the cost-effectiveness of disposable versus reusable products. In a study by Sowell et al. (1987) comparing five methods of incontinence management, disposable pads were the least expensive option and the disposable diaper was the most efficient. Launderable pads were highest in cost, followed by the disposable diaper, staff-managed toileting system, linen service, and disposable pad. The authors noted that supply costs could be reduced by keeping patients dry by toileting them. They also noted that the disposable pad generally was a poor absorbent and had to be changed soon after the incontinent episode.

Hu, Kaltreider, and Igou (1990) investigated the cost-effectiveness and complications of disposable versus reusable diapers in nursing home residents. Residents were randomly assigned to the disposable product or cloth diaper groups. A 4-day baseline of frequency, volume, and type of incontinence was collected. Implementation of the study lasted 5 weeks: the treatment group (n = 34) received disposable diapers and the control group (n = 34) received reusable diapers. The treatment group experienced significant improvement in skin condition when compared to the control group. Also, disposable products provided a cost-savings by eliminating laundry costs. This study used a randomized assignment to intervention groups and a prolonged implementation time to detect changes in skin integrity. However, further research is needed to investigate long-term effects of disposable and reusable product use, the acceptance by patients and staff, and the potential effect of the product on the outcome of other treatment interventions (i.e., behavioral therapies).

IMPLICATIONS FOR NURSING RESEARCH

Incontinence is a complex phenomenon with physiologic, social, and psychologic consequences. Research on the incidence and prevalence of incontinence indicates that different types of incontinence predominate in different groups of individuals. For example, stress incontinence is commonly found in community-dwelling females, but males tend to have urge incontinence. In contrast, females in the long-term care setting have incontinence arising from uninhibited bladder contractions often involving large volume losses. The explanation for the differences is unclear. There may be an interaction between other chronic illnesses that are often present in institutionalized women with dysfunction in urinary elimination that manifests itself in a different type of incontinence seen in the long-term care setting. Research is needed with subgroups of the population such as impaired, older adults living at home or attending medical day care to determine intraindividual and environmental effects on continence status. Studies of incontinence among males and different ethnic groups also are needed.

Research has also revealed that incontinence is not a steady state, that is, remission does occur. Yet little is known regarding remission and whether it is related to changes in the condition of the genitourinary tract or to other factors. The natural history and development of incontinence are not understood. In some adults, large volume losses occur at night: the relationship between nocturnal enuresis and incontinence that occurs during the day needs further exploration. The role of volitional control and motivation to be continent needs further exploration. Some researchers noted that psychologic factors and personality, yet to be measured, may have a role in within-group variability, making findings difficult to interpret. A classification system to measure the severity of incontinence also is needed. Besides the frequency of incontinent episodes and amount of fluid loss, other factors may influence severity such as psychologic impact, the time of day, and antecedent factors to the loss.

There is agreement that a careful history and physical care are required before treatment can be instituted (Agency for Health Care Policy and Research Guidelines [AHCPR], 1991). Yet a disturbing fact is that only half of community-dwelling adults with incontinence seek medical help, and incontinence may be underreported and, therefore, undertreated in the long-term care setting. There is no information regarding the consequences of untreated incontinence. For example, are community-dwelling women with stress incontinence placed on a trajectory of developing the type of incontinence seen in long-term care residents?

Societal attitudes and expectations about aging and incontinence are barriers to receiving effective treatment. Testing methods for increasing help-seeking behaviors is an important focus of nursing research. It is important to note that research most often is conducted with individuals who sought help for incontinence and, therefore, is not representative of all incontinent adults. An essential first step in targeting health promotion strategies is to acquire knowledge about vulnerable individuals. Therefore, efforts must be targeted at adults to seek assistance and treatment for incontinence.

Many studies often lack a control group for comparison. The invasive nature of urodynamic evaluation creates further difficulty in obtaining willing participants. Innovative methods to recruit institutionalized and community-dwelling subjects are needed. Also, the development of valid and reliable noninvasive assessment techniques are needed.

There is no single treatment for incontinence, but the National Institutes of Health Consensus Development Conference (1990) and the AHCPR Guideline on Urinary Incontinence in the Adult (1991) recommended stages of treatment. The least invasive, such as behavioral therapies, is the most preferable initial step. Pharmacologic and surgical interventions can be combined with behavioral ones for complex cases or mixed types of incontinence.

There is research identifying factors that predict successful outcomes of interventions for incontinence. Research is needed to identify the consumers' preferences to treatment strategies and their decisions in selecting one treatment over another. However, more research also is needed, especially regarding the interaction between the individual and the environment. There is evidence of a lack of correlation between subjective reports of severity of incontinence and objective clinical findings, indicating a need for an integrative approach to assessment and treatment (Frazer et al., 1989). Many incontinence treatment strategies are labor intensive. Future research should investigate ways in which the labor intensity can be decreased while effectiveness of outcomes of the treatment remains high.

Nurse practitioners are effective in the assessment and treatment of incontinence (Ouslander, 1986). Continence clinics run by specially trained nurses in the inpatient and outpatient settings should be introduced and evaluated for their impact on patient outcomes and costs of health care. Assessment algorithms are in various stages of development, and further refinement should continue. The identification of outcomes and evaluation of the effectiveness of the nurse practitioner and/or geriatric nurse specialist as the provider of incontinence treatment is crucially needed.

In summary, urinary incontinence is a complex intraindividual disruption of the elimination of urine. Research shows that incontinence is not an inevitable process of aging, and yet many affected individuals do not seek help. The prevalence and type of incontinence differ by setting and gender. Many treatment modalities have been devised. Behavioral therapies show promise for both outpatient and inpatient populations. Replication of intervention studies, especially those with small samples, is recommended.

More nursing research is needed to understand the natural development and remission of incontinence, to identify risk factors to being incontinent, and to match affected adults to the most appropriate and effective treatment. Nurses play a pivotal role in the assessment and treatment of incontinence. The outcomes for nursing interventions must be clearly articulated, and methods to evaluate the effectiveness of the interventions are needed in future nursing research programs.

REFERENCES

Agency for Health Care Policy and Research, 1992. *Urinary incontinence in the adult.* Rockville, MD: Department of Health and Human Services.

Baigis-Smith, J., Smith, D., Rose, M., & Newman, D. (1989). Managing urinary incontinence in community-residing elderly persons. *Gerontologist, 29,* 229–233.

Bates, P., Bradley, W., Glen, G., et al. (1979). The standardization of technology of lower urinary tract function. *Journal of Urology, 121,* 551–554.

Brink, C., Sampselle, C., Wells, T., Diokno, A., & Gillis, G. (1989). A digital test for pelvic floor muscle strength in older women with urinary incontinence. *Nursing Research, 38,* 196–199.

Brocklehurst, J., Andrews, K., Richards, B., & Laycock, P. (1985). Incidence and correlates of incontinence in stroke patients. *Journal of the American Geriatrics Society, 33,* 540–542.

Burgio, K., & Burgio, L. (1986). Behavioral therapies for urinary incontinence in the elderly. *Clinics of Geriatric Medicine, 2,* 809–827.

Burgio, K., & Engel, B. (1987). Urinary incontinence. Behavioral assessment and treatment. In L. Cartensen & B. Edelstein (Eds.) *Handbook of clinical gerontology* (pp. 252–266). New York: Pergamon Press.

Burgio, K., Matthews, K., & Engel, B. (1988, November). Prevalence of urinary incontinence in health perimenopausal women. Paper presented at the meeting of the Gerontological Society of America, San Francisco, CA.

Burgio, K., Whitehead, W., & Engel, B. (1985). Urinary incontinence in the elderly. *Annals of Internal Medicine, 103,* 507–515.

Burgio, K., Stutzman, R., & Engel, B. (1989). Behavioral training for post-prostatectomy urinary incontinence. *Journal of Urology, 141,* 303–306.

Burgio, L., Engel, B., Hawkins, A., McCormick, K., Jones, K., & Scheve, A. (1990). A staff management system for maintaining improvements in continence with elderly nursing home residents. *Journal of Applied Behavioral Analysis, 23,* 111–118.

Burton, J., Pearce, L., Burgio, K., Engel, B., & Whitehead, W. (1988). Behavioral training for urinary incontinence in elderly ambulatory patients. *Journal of the American Geriatrics Society, 36,* 693–698.

Cartensen, L., & Edelstein, B. (Eds.). (1987). *Handbook of clinical gerontology.* New York: Pergamon Press.

Castleden, C., Duffin, H., Asher, M., & Yeomanson, C. (1985). Factors influencing outcome in elderly patients with urinary incontinence and detrusor instability. *Age and Ageing, 14,* 303–307.

Creason, N., Grybowski, J., Burgener, S., Whippo, C., Yeo, S., & Richardson, B. (1989). Prompted voiding therapy for urinary incontinence in aged female nursing home residents. *Journal of Advanced Nursing, 14,* 120–126.

Diokno, A. (1990). Diagnostic categories of incontinence and the role of urodynamic testing. *Journal of the American Geriatrics Society, 38,* 300–305.

Diokno, A., Brown, M., Brock, B., Herzog, A., & Normolle, D. (1988). Clinical and cystometric characteristics of continent and incontinent noninstitutionalized elderly. *Journal of Urology, 140,* 567–571.

Dougherty, M., Abrams, R., & McKey, P. (1986). An instrument to assess the dynamic characteristics of circumvaginal musculature. *Nursing Research, 35,* 202–206.

Ekelund, P., Bergstrom, H., Milsom, I., Norlen, L., & Rignell, S. (1988). Quantification of urinary incontinence in elderly women with the 48 hour pad test. *Archives of Gerontology and Geriatrics, 7,* 281–287.

Engel, B., Burgio, L., McCormick, K., Hawkins, A., Scheve, A., & Leahy, E. (1990). Behavioral treatment of incontinence in the long-term care setting. *Journal of the American Geriatric Society, 38,* 361–363.

Fantl, J. A., Harkins, S., Wyman, J., Choi, S., & Taylor, J. (1987). Fluid loss quantification test in women with urinary incontinence: A test–retest analysis. *Obstetrics & Gynecology, 70,* 739–743.

Fantl, J. A., Wyman, J., McClish, D., Harkins, S., Elswick, R., Taylor, J., & Hadley, E. (1991). Efficacy of bladder training in older women with urinary incontinence. *Journal of the American Medical Association, 265,* 609–613.

Folstein, M., Folstein, S., & McHugh, P. (1975). A practical method for grading the cognitive state of patients for the clinician. *Journal of Psychiatric Research, 12,* 189–198.

Frazer, M., Haylen, B., & Sutherst, J. (1989). The severity of urinary incontinence in women. *British Journal of Urology, 63,* 14–15.

Frazer, M., Sutherst, J., & Holland, E. (1987). Visual analogue scores and urinary incontinence. *British Medical Journal, 295*(6598), 582.

Hadley, E., Abbey, J., Awad, S., Burgio, K., Craighead, W., Diokno, A., Engel, B., Fantl, J. A., Jarvis, G., Mitteness, L., Ory, M., Ouslander, J., Resnick, N., Rooney, V., Schneider, E., Schucker, B., Wells, T., Whitehead, W., Williams, M., & Willington, F. (1986). Bladder training and related therapies for urinary incontinence in older people. *Journal of the American Medical Association, 256,* 372–379.

Harris, T. (1986). Aging in the eighties. Prevalence and impact of urinary problems in individuals age 65 years and over. Washington DC.: *NCHS Advancedata. No. 121.*

Hawkins, A., Langford, A., Engel, B., & Burgio, L. (In review). The effects of supervisory feedback plus contingencies on staff compliance to assigned prompted voids in a geriatric long-term care facility.

Herzog, A., Diokno, A., Brown, M. B., Normolle, D., & Brock, B. (1990). Two year incidence, remission, and change patterns of urinary incontinence in noninstitutionalized older adults. *Journal of Gerontology, 45*(2), 67–74.

Herzog, A., Fultz, N., Brock, B., Brown, M. B., & Diokno, A. (1988). Urinary incontinence and psychological distress among older adults. *Psychology and Aging, 3,* 115–121.

Herzog, A., & Fultz, N. (1988). Urinary incontinence in the community: Prevalence, consequences, management, and beliefs. *Topics in Geriatric Rehabilitation, 3,* 1–12.

Hilton, P. (1987). Urinary incontinence in women. *British Medical Journal, 295*(6595), 425–433.

Hilton, P., & Stanton, S. (1981). Algorithmic method for assessing urinary incontinence in elderly women. *British Medical Journal, 282*(6268), 940–942.

Hu, T. (1990). Impact of urinary incontinence on health-care costs. *Journal of the American Geriatrics Society, 38,* 292–295.

Hu, T., Kaltreider, L., & Igou, J. (1990). The cost effectiveness of disposable versus reusable diapers. *Journal of Gerontological Nursing, 16*(2), 19–24.

Hu, T., Igou, J., Kaltreider, L., Yu, L., Rohner, T., Dennis, P., Craighead, W., Hadley, E., & Ory, M. (1989). A clinical trial of a behavioral therapy on reduced urinary incontinence in nursing homes. *Journal of the American Medical Association, 261,* 2656–2662.

Institute of Medicine (1986). *Improving the quality of care in nursing homes.* Washington DC: National Academy Press.

International Continence Society (1988). The standardization of terminology of lower urinary tract function. *Scandinavian Journal of Urology and Nephrology Supplementum, 114,* 5–19.

Jagger, C., Clarke, M., & Davies, R. (1986). The elderly at home: Indices of disability. *Journal of Epidemiology and Community Health, 40,* 139–142.

Jirovec, M., Brink, C., & Wells, T. (1988). Nursing assessments in the inpatient geriatric populations. *Nursing Clinics of North America, 23,* 219–230.
Kane, R., Ouslander, J., & Abrass, I. (1989). *Essentials of clinical geriatrics.* New York: McGraw Hill.
Kegel, A. (1948). Progressive resistance exercise in the functional restoration of the perineal muscles. *American Journal of Obstetrics and Gynecology, 56,* 238–248.
McCormick, K., & Burgio, K. (1984). Incontinence. An update on nursing care measures. *Journal of Gerontological Nursing, 10*(10), 16–23.
McCormick, K., Scheve, A., & Leahy, E. (1988). Nursing management of urinary incontinence in geriatric inpatients. *Nursing Clinics of North America, 23,* 231–264.
McCormick, K., Burgio, L., Engel, B., Scheve, A., & Leahy, E. (1992). Treating urinary incontinence in nursing home residents: An augmented prompted void approach for the demented. *Journal of Gerontological Nursing, 14*(2), 1–6.
McCormick, K., Cella, M., Scheve, A., & Engel, B. (1990). Cost-effectiveness of treating incontinence in severely mobility-impaired long-term care residents. *Quality Review Bulletin, 16,* 438–443.
McCormick, K., Burgio, L., Scheve, A., Hawkins, A., Leahy, E., & Engel, B. (In review). The effect of changing prompted voiding schedules in the treatment of incontinence in nursing home residents.
Middaugh, S., Whitehead, W., Burgio, K., & Engel, B. (1989). Biofeedback in treatment of urinary incontinence in stroke patients. *Biofeedback and Self Regulation, 14,* 3–19.
Miller, A. (1984). Nurse/patient dependency—a review of different approaches with particular reference to studies of the dependency of elderly patients. *Journal of Advanced Nursing, 9,* 479–486.
Miller, A. (1985). A study of the dependency of elderly patients in wards using different methods of nursing care. *Age and Ageing, 14,* 132–138.
Miller, J. (1990). Assessing urinary incontinence. *Journal of Gerontological Nursing, 16*(3), 15–19.
Mitteness, L. (1987a). So what do you expect when you're 85? Urinary incontinence in late life. In J. Roth & P. Conrad (Eds.), *Research in the sociology of health care.* (Vol. 6, pp. 177–219). Greenwich, CT: JAI Press.
Mitteness, L. (1987b). The management of urinary incontinence by community living elderly. *Gerontologist, 27,* 185–193.
Mohide, E. (1986). The prevalence and scope of urinary incontinence. *Clinics in Geriatric Medicine, 2,* 639–655.
Molander, U., Ekelund, P., Mellstrom, D., Milsom, I., Norlen, L., & Fogelburg, M. (1989). Neurological examination of elderly women under investigation for urinary incontinence. *Archives of Gerontology and Geriatrics, 9,* 77–85.
Morishita, L. (1988). Nursing evaluation and treatment of geriatric outpatients with urinary incontinence: Geriatric day hospital model: A case study. *Nursing Clinics of North America, 23,* 189–206.
National Institutes of Health Consensus Development Conference (1990). Urinary incontinence in adults. *Journal of the American Geriatrics Society, 38,* 265–272.
Norberg, A., Sandstrom, S., Norberg, B., Eriksson, S., & Sandman, P. (1984). The urine smell around patients with urinary incontinence. *Gerontology, 30,* 261–266.
Norton, C. (1982). The effects of urinary incontinence in women. *International Rehabilitation Medicine, 4,* 9–14.

O'Donnell, P., Beck, C., & Walls, R. (1990). Serial incontinence assessment in elderly inpatient males. *Journal of Rehabilitation Research, 27,* 1–8.

Ouslander, J. (1986). Diagnostic evaluation of geriatric incontinence. *Clinics of Geriatric Medicine, 2,* 715–730.

Ouslander, J. (1989). Assessment and treatment of incontinence in the nursing home. In P. Katz & E. Calkins (Eds.), *Principles and practices of nursing home care* (pp. 247–274). New York: Springer Publishing Co.

Ouslander, J. (1990). Urinary incontinence in nursing homes. *Journal of the American Geriatrics Society, 38,* 289–291.

Ouslander, J., Blaustein, J., Connor, A., & Pitt, A. (1988). Habit training and oxybutynin for incontinence in nursing home patients: A placebo-controlled trial. *Journal of the American Geriatrics Society, 36,* 40–46.

Ouslander, J., Greengold, B., & Chen, S. (1987). External catheter use and urinary tract infections among incontinent male nursing home patients. *Journal of the American Geriatrics Society, 35,* 1063–1070.

Ouslander, J., Urman, H., & Uman, G. (1986). Development and testing of an incontinence monitoring record. *Journal of the American Geriatric Society, 34,* 83–90.

Palmer, M., McCormick, K., & Langford, A. (1989). Do nurses consistently document incontinence? *Journal of Gerontological Nursing, 15*(12), 11–16.

Pannill, F., Williams, T., & Davis, R. (1988). Evaluation and treatment of urinary incontinence in long term care. *Journal of the American Geriatrics Society, 36,* 902–910.

Parkin, D., & Davis, J. (1986). Use of a visual analogue scale in the diagnosis of urinary incontinence. *British Medical Journal, 293*(6543), 365–366.

Petrilli, C., Traughber, B., & Schnelle, J. (1988). Behavioral management in the inpatient geriatric population. *Nursing Clinics of North America, 23,* 265–277.

Petrucci, K., McCormick, K., & Scheve, A. (1987). Documenting patient care needs: Do nurses do it? *Journal of Gerontological Nursing, 13*(11), 34–38.

Pieper, B., Cleland, V., Johnson, D., O'Reilly, J. (1989). Inventing urine incontinence devices for women. *Image: Journal of Nursing Scholarship, 21,* 205–209.

Resnick, N., Yalla, S., & Laurino, E. (1989). The pathophysiology of urinary incontinence among institutionalized elderly persons. *The New England Journal of Medicine, 320,* 1–7.

Roe, B. (1990). Study of the effects of education on patients' knowledge and acceptance of their indwelling urethral catheters. *Journal of Advanced Nursing, 15,* 223–231.

Roe, B., & Brocklehurst, J. (1987). Study of patients with indwelling catheters. *Journal of Advanced Nursing, 12,* 713–718.

Roth, J., & Conrad, P. (Eds.). (1987). *Research in the sociology of health care* (Vol. 6). Greenwich, CT: JAI Press.

Schnelle, J. (1991). *Managing urinary incontinence in the elderly.* New York: Springer Publishing Co.

Schnelle, J., Sowell, V., Hu, T., & Traughber, B. (1988). Reduction of urinary incontinence in nursing homes: Does it reduce or increase costs? *Journal of the American Geriatrics Society, 36,* 34–39.

Schnelle, J., Traughber, B., Sowell, V., Newman, D., Petrilli, C., & Ory, M. (1989). Prompted voiding treatment of urinary incontinence in nursing home patients. A behavioral management approach for nursing home staff. *Journal of the American Geriatrics Society, 37,* 1051–1057.

Sommer, P., Nielsen, K., Bauer, T., Kristensen, E., Hermann, G., Steven, K., & Nordling, J. (1990). Voiding patterns in men evaluated by a questionnaire survey. *British Journal of Urology, 65,* 155–160.

Sowell, V., Schnelle, J., Hu, T., & Traughber, B. (1987). A cost comparison of five methods of managing urinary incontinence. *Quality Review Bulletin, 13,* 411–414.

Starer, P., & Libow, L. (1988). The measurement of residual urine in the evaluation of incontinent nursing home residents. *Archives of Gerontology and Geriatrics, 7,* 75–81.

Voith, A. (1988). Alterations in urinary elimination: Concepts, research, and practice. *Rehabilitation Nursing, 13,* 122–131.

Warren, J. (1986). Catheters and catheter care. *Clinics in Geriatric Medicine, 2,* 857–871.

Watson, R. (1989). A nursing trial of urinary sheath systems on male hospitalized patients. *Journal of Advanced Nursing, 14,* 467–470.

Wein, A. (1986). Physiology of micturition. *Clinics in Geriatric Medicine, 2,* 689–699.

Wells, T. (1980). Promoting urine control in older adults. *Geriatric Nursing, 1,* 236–240.

Wells, T. (1988). Additional treatments for urinary incontinence. *Topics in Geriatric Rehabilitation, 3,* 48–57.

Wells, T., Brink, C., & Diokno, A. (1987). Urinary incontinence in elderly women: Clinical findings. *Journal of the American Geriatric Society, 35,* 933–939.

Wells, T., & Diokno, A. (1989). Urinary incontinence in the elderly. *Seminars in Neurology, 9,* 60–67.

Worth, A., Dougherty, M., & McKey, P. (1986). Development and testing of the circumvaginal muscles rating scale. *Nursing Research, 35,* 166–168.

Wyman, J. (1988). Nursing assessment of the incontinent geriatric outpatient population. *Nursing Clinics of North America, 23,* 169–187.

Wyman, J., Choi, S., Harkins, S., Wilson, M., & Fantl, J. A. (1988). The urinary diary in evaluation of incontinent women: A test–retest analysis. *Obstetrics and Gynecology, 71,* 812–817.

Wyman, J., Harkins, S., Choi, S., Taylor, J., & Fantl, J. A. (1987). Psychosocial impact of urinary incontinence in women. *Obstetrics and Gynecology, 70,* 378–381.

Wyman, J., Harkins, S., & Fantl, J. A. (1990). Psychological impact of urinary incontinence in the community-dwelling population. *Journal of the American Geriatrics Society, 38,* 282–288.

Yu, L. (1987). Incontinence stress index: Measuring psychological impact. *Journal of Gerontological Nursing, 13,* 18–25.

Yu, L., Kaltreider, L., Hu, T., Igou, J., & Craighead, W. (1989). The ISQ-P tool measuring stress associated with incontinence. *Journal of Gerontological Nursing, 15,* 9–15.

Chapter 3

Diabetes Mellitus

EDNA HAMERA
SCHOOL OF NURSING
UNIVERSITY OF KANSAS MEDICAL CENTER

CONTENTS

Diabetes mellitus is a major health problem in the United States. Approximately 5.8 million people have been diagnosed by a physician, and an additional 4 to 5 million have diabetes but have yet to be diagnosed (National Diabetes Data Group, 1985). Health care of individuals with diabetes is demanding and complex. Although nurses are essential to the acute and long-term care of individuals with diabetes, only a few are involved in research related to diabetes. In this review, nursing research on diabetes mellitus published during the past decade is examined to identify strengths and weaknesses in the research and to project future research needs. Studies prior to 1980 were not included because many were focused on topics that are not a major part of current nursing practice.

A decision was made to focus on published studies because of the difficulty in accessing unpublished work. Studies were included in which investigators focused on chronic illness and included subjects with diabetes as a subsample. Evaluation of educational programs for health professionals who care for individuals with diabetes, studies involving animal prototypes (or animal models), and studies of the parents of children with diabetes were excluded. Research on pregnant women with diabetes was excluded because these studies were focused on high-risk mothers and infants, a separate area. Furthermore, studies of pregnancy and diabetes often contain both women with diabetes who became pregnant and women who develop the symptom of diabetes during pregnancy.

In an initial hand search of the major nursing research journals, *Nursing Research; Research in Nursing and Health; Image; Journal of Nursing Scholarship; Advances in Nursing Science; International Journal of Nursing Research; Journal of Advanced Nursing;* and *Western Journal of Nursing Research,* 19 full-length studies were found, and three of these were studies of chronic illness that included a subsample with diabetes. A *Cumulative Index to Nursing and Allied Health Literature* computer search was done to check for any research that may have been missed.

In addition to nursing research journals, two diabetes journals in which nursing research frequently is published, *Diabetes Care* and *The Diabetes Educator,* were searched. *Diabetes Care* began listing the credentials of authors in 1983, so from 1980 to 1983 information contained in the articles was used to determine if the authors were nurses. *The Diabetes Educator* was first published in 1983. Because the focus of this review is nurse-led research, studies selected from these sources were limited to those in which the first author was a nurse. Twenty-seven studies were found in the two diabetes journals. Thus, from all sources, there were 46 articles attributed to nurse investigators.

Prior to review of specific studies, the definitions used throughout this review are clarified. The conceptual frameworks (or lack of them) are summarized and issues about scientific methods highlighted. The critical review of selected studies is followed by a summary and discussion of future research.

DEFINITIONS

An important distinction in diabetes is insulin-dependent diabetes mellitus (IDDM), which constitutes about 5–10% of all individuals with diabetes, and noninsulin-dependent diabetes mellitus (NIDDM), which comprises the remainder of individuals with diabetes. The distinction between these two types of diabetes is important in clinical characteristics, management, and prognosis. IDDM usually emerges in children and is characterized by the absence of endogenous insulin. NIDDM usually emerges in adulthood and is characterized by a decrease in sensitivity to endogenous insulin. Although both types have a familial component, the genetic transmission is much higher in NIDDM than in IDDM and appears to vary among ethnic groups. In the United States the prevalence of NIDDM is higher in blacks, Mexican Americans, and Native Americans (Bennett, 1990). NIDDM is also associated with obesity, parity, a sedentary life style, and aging. The major clinical goal for individuals with NIDDM is often weight reduction. In contrast, weight loss in individuals with IDDM, who are not usually overweight, may indicate poor control. Making the distinction between these two types of diabetes has not been easy. Currently, the most acceptable method is evaluation of beta-cell functioning by C-peptide levels (Madsbad, 1990). C-peptide concentrations are an indicator of endogenous insulin secretory capacity. Although most of the nurse investigators who have conducted recent research differentiate between IDDM and NIDDM, they often do not report the criteria used in making the distinction.

Related to the problem of distinguishing between types of diabetes is the measurement of how well the diabetes state is being controlled in the affected individual. Brown (1988) discussed this issue in her review of patient teaching interventions and concluded that the best single indicator is glycosylated hemoglobin. Glycosylated hemoglobin is the joining of hemoglobin and glucose. Specifically, hemoglobin becomes glycosylated in red blood cells in proportion to an individual's average serum blood glucose level. This glycosylation is nonreversible and therefore lasts as long as the life of the red blood cell, which is about 120 days. Thus glycosylated hemoglobin level reflects a time-averaged blood glucose concentration over the previous 4 to 8 weeks (Gabbay, 1976; Nathan, Singer, Hurxthal, & Goodson, 1984). A single indicator may not be a valid measure of diabetic control. Some nurse researchers (Edelstein & Linn, 1987; Pollock, 1989) have used a combination of indices (e.g., triglycerides and neuropathy) and weighted them to form a global measure of metabolic control; however, the rational for the selection of these indices and their weighting was not reported.

CONCEPTUAL BASES OF STUDIES

A conceptual basis or framework was identified in only 15 of the 46 studies reviewed. The lack of inclusion of a conceptual basis in some of the studies may have been due to lack of space in some of the journals. Most of the frameworks identified were applied or adapted from the behavioral or biological sciences. Havlin and Cryer (1987) clinically tested physiologic theories explaining the night-to-morning increase in blood glucose levels in diabetes. Four researchers utilized social learning theory as their conceptual framework (Alogna, 1980; Edelstein & Linn, 1987; Massouh, Steele, Alseth, & Diekmann, 1989; Schlenk & Hart, 1984). Bloom-Cerkoney and Hart (1980) and Given, Given, Gallin, and Condon (1983) used the health belief model to guide their research. In one nurse-led program of diabetes research, investigators adapted frameworks from the behavioral sciences (Fox et al., 1984; Hamera et al., 1988; O'Connell et al., 1984; O'Connell, Hamera, Schorfheide, & Guthrie, 1990). The investigators of this program developed and tested a symptom self-regulation model in diabetes adapted from a self-control theory and a model of illness representation.

Several studies used nursing conceptual frameworks or theories. Pollock (1986, 1989) used Roy's nursing model for her guiding framework, but the concepts in Pollock's model of adaptation to diabetes mellitus were derived from stress-adaptation models. Two groups of nurse researchers employed exclusively Orem's nursing theory as the basis for their studies (Frey & Denyes, 1989; Germain & Nemchik, 1988). Germain and Nemchik used Orem's theory only as a broad framework, whereas Frey and Denyes actually tested hypotheses derived from Orem's self-care theory.

SCIENTIFIC METHODS

The studies were reviewed systematically for clarity of purpose and/or research questions, size and specification of sample, reliability and validity of instruments, adequacy of design in addressing the purpose or research questions, appropriateness of statistics, and congruence of findings with conclusions. The most obvious methodologic problem in diabetes research conducted by nurses and other health professionals is the use of instruments with little or no established reliability and validity. Each diabetes treatment center appears to generate its own instruments to measure diabetes knowledge, self-care, and compliance. Also, researchers who have administered interviews have failed either to assess or to report interviewing and coding reliability.

The majority of studies (n = 42) identified were nonexperimental. Almost all researchers utilized convenience samples. The sample sizes frequently were small; 13 of the studies had 30 or fewer subjects. With a few exceptions, nurse researchers have not addressed the representativeness of their samples. Most nurse researchers specified research questions but a few investigators did not address the questions in the results or discussion of the report. Univariate statistics frequently were used when the purpose and research question dictated multivariate statistics. In several studies in which multivariate statistics were employed, the sample size was not sufficient to yield reliable results. These methodologic problems occurred more frequently in the 28 studies led by baccalaureate or master's prepared nurses.

CRITICAL REVIEW OF SELECTED STUDIES

The nursing research on diabetes during the last decade can be classified into studies of: (a) epidemiology (n = 1); (b) self-care technology (n = 13); (c) physiologic studies of complications (n = 3); (d) perceptions of diabetes and the diabetic regimen (n = 11); (e) social-psychologic factors, compliance, and metabolic control (n = 16); and (f) evaluations of nursing interventions (n = 2). One of the studies in the last category involved a meta analysis evaluating the effects of diabetes education. Two seminal diabetes studies will be briefly discussed before reviewing the selected studies.

Seminal Studies

Two studies that frequently are cited as landmark studies of compliance were conducted by nurses. Watkins and colleagues (Watkins, Roberts, Williams, Martin, & Coyle, 1967a) from the University of North Carolina at Chapel Hill shared their findings from a large study of patients with diabetes. During interviews and observations of patients (N = 162) in their homes, the investigators examined the extent of insulin and oral hypoglycemic medication errors. They reported that 58% of the subgroup taking insulin (n = 115) made some type of medication error, involving either the incorrect measurement of insulin or a misunderstanding of the insulin prescription. Errors in medication increased with duration of diabetes and with dissatisfaction with medical care. Of the subsample (n = 47) of individuals on oral hypoglycemic agents, 26% made medication errors. Follow-up interviews were conducted 12 to 18 months later with equivalent findings.

Utilizing a subgroup from the sample used in previous work (Watkins et al., 1967a), Watkins and colleagues (Watkins, Williams, Martin, Hogan, & Anderson, 1967b) examined the relationships among what individuals with diabetes know, what they do, and diabetic control. Five aspects of diabetes management were explored in 60 individuals using insulin. The areas of management explored were insulin administration, insulin dosage, urine testing, meals and meal spacing, and foot care. In addition, patients' general knowledge of diabetes was assessed. The researchers reported that approximately half of the subjects had unacceptable management in four or five areas. Those who had more knowledge about diabetes had better management. Disease control, measured by physicians' rating of progress notes and laboratory values from subjects' medical records, was not related to diabetes management.

Although the investigators did not present psychometric properties for their measures of diabetes knowledge and management, and their measure of diabetes control would be unacceptable by current standards, these studies and others from the group (Williams, Anderson, Watkins, Coyle, 1967; Williams, Martin, Hogan, Watkins, & Ellis, 1967) frequently are cited to support the lack of compliance in individuals with diabetes. The work of Watkins and colleagues continues to be cited because: (a) the sample was recruited from multiple sources, thereby increasing its representativeness; (b) the areas of self-care examined continue to be clinically relevant; and (c) the interviews and observations were conducted in patients' homes, thereby increasing their validity.

Epidemiology

Only one study that addressed epidemiologic issues was identified. Kahn, Marshall, Baxter, Shetterly, and Hamman (1990) identified 20 individuals from clinical records: 10 (5 Hispanic and 5 white) with abnormal glucose tolerance tests, and 10 (5 Hispanic and 5 white) with normal glucose tolerance tests. The researchers contacted subjects' family members to determine if family members accurately reported their family history of diabetes and to determine if those who had a positive family history were more likely to be screened for diabetes than those who had a negative family history. One hundred ninety-seven relatives of the 20 patients were interviewed. There were no differences in accuracy of reporting family history by relatives of patients with and without diabetes. Relatives with a positive family history of diabetes were more likely to know about screening for diabetes. Relatives who were Hispanic and had a positive family history of diabetes were more likely to be screened than Hispanics with a negative family history. No differences were found in the rate of screening between relatives who were white who had positive and negative family histories. The investigators expressed concern about the low rate of screening of relatives who had positive family histories for NIDDM (29% for whites and 33% for Hispanic).

This is the only nurse-led study designed to investigate ethnic differences and diabetes. Because there is a higher prevalence of NIDDM diabetes in black, Hispanic, and Native American populations, this is an important factor for nurses to study. The Kahn et al. (1990) study also is unique from the others identified in this review in that its focus was on early detection.

Self-care Technology

Technologic advances have made available methods that are more accurate to monitor and manage diabetes mellitus, and nurses have examined the use and effectiveness of these methods. The majority of the 13 studies on self-care technology ($n = 10$) were focused on patients' use of blood glucose self-monitoring, which became available in the late 1970s. Other studies in this category ($n = 3$) included an investigation of patient use of continuous subcutaneous insulin infusion therapy (Guinn, Bailey, & Mecklenburg, 1988), and the multiple usage of insulin syringes by patients (Poteet, Reinert, & Ptak, 1987; Turner & Lancaster, 1984).

With the technologic advancements in assessing blood glucose, nurse researchers addressed: (a) the accuracy of visual reading of reagent strips (Auerhahn, Bergman, Kumar, & Morgan, 1985; Barr, Leichter, & Taylor, 1984); (b) the stability of reagent strips (Freeman, 1986; Wakefield, Wilberding, Wakefield, Booth, & Buckwalter, 1989); and (c) the agreement among various reflectance meters developed to read reagent strips and the accuracy of these blood glucose readings with standard laboratory methods (Ahern, Bates, & Tamborlane, 1988; Fairclough, Clements, Filer, & Bell, 1983; Giordano et al., 1989; Gifford-Jorgensen et al., 1986). One group of researchers conducted an experimental study with volunteers, of whom only 21% had diabetes, to examine the ease of learning to perform blood glucose monitoring with four different meters (Jenkins, Powers, & Molitch, 1988). One researcher (Saucier, 1984) hypothesized that blood glucose self-monitoring would improve metabolic control. Using an ex post facto design, the hypothesis was not supported. This hypothesis also has been tested by other health professionals and, as in this study, usually has not been supported.

Investigations of patients' use of technologic advances have been led almost exclusively by master's or baccalaureate prepared clinicians, who have not articulated any conceptual basis for their work. Although the findings are often clinically applicable, their relevance becomes outdated as technology advances. Consideration of the broader issue of patients' perception, use of the products of technologic advances, and use of conceptual frameworks to understand how patients adapt to and are changed by these products is absent.

Three studies in this category, self-care technology, merit description in more detail. Noting that patients with diabetes may reuse insulin syringes,

Turner and Lancaster (1984) investigated the frequency of reuse, demographic characteristics, aseptic self-administration techniques, and rates of injection site inflammation in individuals who reuse insulin syringes. Subjects were interviewed regarding their practices in the preceeding 5 years. Aseptic self-administration of insulin was measured by a rating scale, and inflammation sites were measured by self-report and validated by chart review. The investigators stated that 44.4% of the subjects reported reusing their syringes. Individuals who reused syringes were older and had been using insulin longer; black individuals were more likely than white individuals to reuse syringes. Only a small percentage of the sample (10%) experienced an inflammation. The large sample (N = 302) and similarity of the sample with a national sample of diabetics supports the generalizability of the findings. However, the safety of reusing insulin syringes was not adequately addressed because the data on inflammation sites were derived from patient recall rather than from direct observation. The limited description of the statistical analyses of data made it difficult to assess whether the data were appropriately analyzed.

Poteet et al. (1987) also investigated the frequency and safety of reusing syringes in 166 insulin-dependent diabetics. Using a self-administered questionnaire, they found a percentage of subjects reusing syringes (45%) similar to the percentage reported by Turner and Lancaster (1984). Individuals who reused syringes had the following characteristics; (a) they gave themselves significantly more injections per day, (b) they were more often female, and (c) they were more likely to have a yearly income under $10,000. The investigators reported that there were no differences in preparation for injection between reusers and nonreusers, but it was not clear how this similarity was assessed. The investigators also evaluated safety of syringe reuse by gathering and culturing the syringes of a random sample of 44 subjects who gave themselves more than one injection per day. No pathogenic organisms were isolated, but four syringes were found to be contaminated with normal skin flora compared to none cultured on 44 sterile syringes. Culturing the syringes provided a more sensitive measure of the safety of reuse than did the previous study (Turner & Lancaster, 1984), in which subjects were asked to recall inflammation at injection sites. Poteet and colleagues concluded that the practice of reusing syringes might be safe for some patients.

A more recent study (Wakefield et al., 1989) was undertaken to evaluate the practice of patients' cutting reagent strips longitudinally and using only one half each time that they monitored their blood glucose level. An experimental design was employed to investigate differences in five methods of using reagent strips. The methods involved bisecting strips under sterile and unsterile conditions compared to strips used according to manufacturer's directions. The investigators found no significant differences between the strip conditions. Thus, depending on the patients' vision in reading reagent strips and their dexterity in cutting them, the practice might be reliably used by patients who do not have reflectance meters. This study was well designed and executed except that the nurses were not blind to which strips came from which subjects, a limitation the investigators recognized.

Physiologic Studies of Complications

Three physiologic studies of diabetic complications were identified (Coonrod et al., 1989; Havlin & Cryer, 1987; Hite, 1982). Coonrod et al. (1989) examined a new clinical laboratory test to detect urinary albumin concentrations, an indicator of diabetic nephropathy. The study was well designed and executed.

Hite (1982) examined the relationship between renal threshold for glucose in diabetics and age, gender, type of diabetes, and duration of diabetes in 40 hospitalized subjects. Serum glucose was compared to urine glucose on 423 double- and 410 triple-voided urine specimens. Regression analysis was used to examine the relationship between the variability in the negative boundary of renal threshold (i.e., the individual's highest serum glucose concentration associated with glucosuria) for the double-voided urine, and age, gender, race, duration and type of diabetes, units of insulin prescribed, and creatinine level. Together these variables accounted for 33% of the variance but alone none explained a significant proportion of the variance in renal threshold. Because the majority of subjects' serum glucose was over 200 mg/dl before glucose appeared in the urine, Hite concluded that renal threshold should be checked before patients use urine glucose testing to adjust insulin dosages. Unfortunately, the relevance of Hite's findings are dated. With the ease and availability of blood glucose self-monitoring, urine glucose testing is rapidly being replaced by blood glucose testing.

Havlin and Cryer (1987) evaluated serum glucose on specimens collected three times during the night from 75 hospitalized diabetics to evaluate whether the hypothesized somogyi and dawn phenomena proposed to explain morning hyperglycemia could be supported. The investigators precisely defined the dawn phenomenon as an increment in blood glucose from 3 A.M. to 7 A.M. and the somogyi phenomenon as hyperglycemia after a 3 A.M. blood glucose of less than or equal to 50 mg/dL. The dawn phenomenon occurred in 37% of all profiles (216 profiles), whereas the somogyi phenomenon was detected in only 7% of the profiles. The results were similar for NIDDM and IDDM groups. These findings cannot be generalized to diabetics in other settings, but this study is a good example of clinical application of physiologic theories. The findings illustrated the relatively low incidence of these phenomena in hospitalized patients.

Knowledge, Perceptions, and Attitudes about Diabetes

A number of nurses have conducted descriptive studies to explore: (a) patients' knowledge (Teza, Davis, & Hiss, 1988); (b) perceptions of diabetes and the diabetic regimen (Daschner, 1986; D'Eramo-Melkus & Demas, 1989; Fox et al., 1984; Germain & Nemchik, 1988; Lockwood, Frey, Gladish, & Hiss, 1986; Wierenga, Browning, & Mahn, 1990; Wikblad, Wibell, & Montin, 1990); (c) perceptions of complications (Klosiewski, 1984; Nyhlin, 1990); and (d) perceptions of well-being (Lundman, Asplund, & Norberg, 1990). Many of the investigators did not address the representativeness of their sample or the measurement properties of their questionnaires and interviews. Selected studies that were judged to have more relevance to future research are discussed in more detail.

Germain and Nemchik (1988) developed a self-administered questionnaire to determine the extent to which individuals with diabetes desired to continue self-management if they were hospitalized and the event to which self-management was possible for those who had been hospitalized. Self-management activities included testing urine and blood glucose, selecting diet, taking diabetes pills, preparing and administering insulin, and treating insulin reactions. The sample of 72 individuals with diabetes was recruited from a local American Diabetic Association (ADA) chapter. Approximately 66% of the sample expressed a wish to care for themselves in the hospital. Subjects who had been hospitalized reported that, in most instances, self-management activities were performed by hospital staff. The participants' greatest concern regarding future hospitalization was fear of an insulin reaction with no access to food. The investigators reported that some subjects expressed concern that health professionals in the hospital might not be competent to care for their diabetes. The investigators acknowledged that the sample was not representative because a high proportion were ADA members and therefore may be more compliant with a diabetic regimen. However, the Germain and Nemchik (1988) study raises additional research questions that are important for nurses to address such as what the effect of self-care is on anxiety during hospitalization.

Nyhlin (1990) conducted a study of complications using grounded theory methodology with 14 individuals with IDDM at the time they first developed signs of retinopathy, often the first vascular complication of diabetes. Participants were interviewed at the onset of the disease and 5 years later to determine the coping strategies they used to deal with diabetic complications. Nyhlin concluded that participants generally were successful in coping with complications and identified three overlapping stages in managing complications, which were labeled coming to terms, keeping going, and making sense. Although the investigator did not report any intercoder reliability or conduct participant observation, which is integral to grounded theory methodology, the longitudinal design added a new perspective to understanding the coping process.

The final study (Lundman et al., 1990) in this section was a mail survey of 215 individuals with IDDM who had no severe long-term complications. Subjects were asked to complete a questionnaire of their subjective feeling of well-being on a semantic differential scale developed by the investigators and to rate their experience of having diabetes. The 192 subjects (89%) who returned the questionnaire reported overall positive attitudes about having diabetes. The need to maintain regularity in daily activities and diet management were the greatest problems and retinopathy was rated the complication that caused the greatest concern.

The investigators are to be commended for their attention to the psychometric properties of the well-being scale, although validity data are needed. The investigators' focus on wellness was a contrast to most of the other studies reviewed. Future studies examining perception of diabetes should incorporate positive as well as negative aspects, which may lead to a more accurate representation of the experience. Perception of positive aspects may in fact be one indicator of successful adaptation.

Social-psychologic Factors, Compliance, and Metabolic Control

Studies of the bivariate relationship between locus of control and disease outcome have waned as multivariate models have been proposed in an effort to understand treatment compliance and disease control. Multivariate designs require large samples. A major limitation of many of the studies in this section was the small sample size.

Lundman, Asplund, and Norberg (1988) investigated the construct of tedium and its relationship to perception about diabetes and regimen-related behaviors. Two studies were found in which the relationship of locus of control and metabolic control in diabetes was studied (Edelstein & Linn, 1987; Meize-Grochowski, 1990). In four studies, investigators examined variables in a health belief model (Alogna, 1980; Bloom-Cerkoney & Hart, 1980; Given et al., 1983; & Schlenk & Hart, 1984). Two of the studies (Bloom-Cerkoney & Hart, 1980; Schlenk & Hart, 1984) that focused on factors in a particular health belief model and compliance had sample sizes of 30, an insufficient number to establish reliable relationships.

Given and associates (1983) developed a scale to measure variables in a health belief model. The original 76 items were hypothesized to represent 12 concepts and were administered to 156 individuals with diabetes. Factor analytic methods yielded six clusters: (a) control of effects of diabetes, (b) barriers to diet, (c) social support for diet, (d) barriers to taking medication,

(e) impact of job on therapy, and (f) commitment to benefits of therapy. The clear conceptual base and systematic methodology used in developing this scale is noteworthy.

Alogna (1980) predicted that compliant, noninsulin-dependent obese individuals with diabetes would perceive their disease as more severe and would be more internally controlled. Compliance was defined by amount of weight loss in the previous 3 years and by the level of one blood glucose reading. In a sample of 50, mostly black, female subjects, Alogna reported that subjects in the compliant group perceived their diabetes as being more severe but were not more internally controlled than subjects in the noncompliant group. The investigator noted that a causal relationship could not be inferred, but the results suggested that perceived severity is related to compliance.

The work of other investigators reviewed in this category involved testing nurse-developed or adapted models to understand individuals with diabetes. Frey and Denyes (1989) tested hypotheses regarding the distinction between universal self-care, that is, general self-care actions such as eating a balanced diet, and health deviation self-care, that is, being aware and attending to effects of diabetes [as in Orem's (1991) model]. Thirty-seven adolescents with Type I diabetes completed instruments measuring universal self-care, health deviation self-care, health, control of pathology, and basic conditioning factors. Basic conditioning factors included demographic and socioeconomic factors, as well as health symptoms measured by the Brief Symptom Inventory (Derogatis & Melisarotos, 1983). Although only preliminary measurement data were available on the instruments measuring aspects of Orem's theory, the investigators identified the need for careful evaluation of the instruments. From the findings, universal self-care practices were found to be related to health deviation self-care practices. However, only universal self-care practices were related to selected basic conditioning factors (age and health symptoms). Younger children engaged in more universal self-care practices than older children, and children with fewer health symptoms engaged in fewer universal self-care practices than children with more health symptoms. Health deviation self-care practices were related to control of pathology as measured by metabolic control (glycosylated hemoglobin). The findings must be considered preliminary due to the small sample size, but further research applying Orem's theory to diabetes may help nurses understand how individuals with a chronic disease manage their self-care needs.

Pollock (1989) tested a model of physiologic adaptation in diabetes adapted from Roy's nursing model and the model of researchers studying stress and coping. Individuals' appraisals of their diabetes constituted the focal stimulus, coping styles and demographic variables constituted the contextual stimuli, and hardiness was the residual stimulus. Using multiple regression, measures of five of the variables (outcome stress appraisals, mixed-focus coping patterns, hardiness, patient education, and emotion-focused coping) predicted 56% of the variance in physiologic control. The small sample size ($N = 30$) cast doubt on the reproducibility of the findings, but the investigator's conceptual framework and measure of physiologic control are noteworthy. Pollock measured physiologic control by weighting then summing seven criteria: three biochemical indices and four assessment values obtained from subjects' medical records.

A limitation of the studies reviewed in this section was the lack of follow-up work replicating and extending the findings. A series of studies (Hamera et al., 1988; O'Connell et al., 1984; & O'Connell et al., 1990) led by nurse investigators in the Midwest were conducted to evaluate a model of self-regulation of symptoms in diabetes. From the self-regulation model, the investigators proposed that individuals monitor their disease status by comparing their current state with their standard of well-being. When a discrepancy is experienced and associated with a change in blood glucose, action is taken to relieve the symptom and thereby regulate blood glucose. In a preliminary study conducted to test the model (O'Connell et al., 1984), 38 individuals with Type II diabetes were interviewed to determine whether or not they used symptoms as indicators of blood glucose levels. Thirty (84%) of the sample identified symptoms for one or more blood glucose levels, and 73% of these 30 subjects reported taking actions when the symptoms were present. Those taking actions had better metabolic control as measured by glycosylated hemoglobin levels. Replicating these findings with a sample of 173 individuals with Type II diabetes, Hamera and colleagues (1988) found that a comparable percentage of subjects associated symptoms with blood glucose levels (85%) and took actions when symptoms were present. Approximately 77% took action when they thought their blood glucose was elevated and 89% took action when they thought it was lowered. In this larger study, the investigators found no relationship between associating symptoms with blood glucose levels and taking action and metabolic control as measured by glycosylated hemoglobin levels. Only gender and insulin use were related to symptom association and action taking. Females were more likely than males to report associating symptoms with both high and low blood glucose levels and to report taking action when they experienced these symptoms. Subjects currently using insulin were more likely to associate symptoms with both high and low blood glucose levels than subjects who had previously used insulin. Also, subjects on insulin were more likely to associate symptoms with low blood glucose than subjects on noninsulin treatment regimens.

A natural extension of this research was to examine the accuracy of subjects' blood glucose symptom beliefs and to determine if symptom accuracy was related to metabolic control (O'Connell et al. 1990). To estimate accuracy, 56 subjects completed a symptom checklist composed of their specific symptom blood glucose beliefs and symptoms commonly associated with blood glucose levels. The subjects checked their actual blood glucose level using reagent strips and reflectance meters at random times four times daily for 10 days. Within-subject correlations between symptom ratings and blood glucose levels revealed that subjects' specific symptom beliefs were largely unrelated to actual blood glucose levels. Subjects who had more accurate symptom beliefs for low blood glucose had better metabolic control on two of the three indices of metabolic control: glycosylated hemoglobin levels and the average blood glucose level for the 10 days of the study. Although 88% of the subjects had at least one significant correlation between one of the symptoms commonly associated with high or low blood glucose levels and actual blood glucose, the investigators concluded that these correlations were not large enough to be clinically significant.

The investigators (Hamera et al., 1988; O'Connell et al., 1984; O'Connell et al., 1990) of the self-regulation in diabetes research validated that subjects in their studies had NIDDM by measuring C-peptide levels. Many nurse researchers either have not reported how they differentiated between subjects with Type II diabetes or have used readily available, but inadequate, criteria to distinguish between types of diabetes. Differentiation between Type I and Type II diabetes is important because the clinical goals, management, and prognoses are different. The strength of this program of research on self-regulation of symptoms in diabetes was the careful testing of the model. The investigators concluded that clinicians need to be aware of patients' reliance on symptoms in making decisions about actions to lower or increase their blood glucose and encourage patients to check symptom beliefs by testing actual blood glucose levels when the symptoms are present. The weakness in this program of research was failure of the researchers to explicate the relationship between their self-regulation model and metabolic control.

The investigators of one study (Pieper, Kushion, & Gaida, 1990) examined the effect of having diabetes on one's marriage and spouse. An adapted version of the Beliefs about Diabetes Scale (Given et al., 1983) and a marital adjustment scale were administered to 20 couples. The internal consistency of several subscales in the Beliefs about Diabetes Scale were adequate and appropriately omitted from analysis. Greater perceived barriers to taking medication and to following a diet were positively correlated with higher marital adjustment in the spouse with diabetes. Beliefs about benefits of the diet and marital adjustment were positively correlated in the spouse without diabetes. The findings are preliminary due to the small sample used in this study, but this is an important area that needs attention. Family beliefs about diabetes and family support of individuals with diabetes also may vary by ethnic group.

Three studies were identified in which investigators examined social psychologic variables in chronic illness groups, including a subsample with diabetes (Burckhardt, Woods, Schultz, & Ziebarth, 1989; Pollock, 1986; Primomo, Yates, & Woods, 1990). The samples usually were larger in these studies and therefore adequate for multivariate analysis. The subsamples with diabetes were not large enough to determine reliable similarities and differences from other chronic illness groups. Burckhardt et al. (1989) evaluated the reliability and validity of a quality of life scale for four chronic illness groups. Primomo et al (1990) described social networks and examined the relationship between type and source of support and psychosocial adaptation. Pollock (1986) examined the relationship of hardiness to physiologic and psychologic adaptation in a sample of 60 individuals with diabetes mellitus, rheumatoid arthritis, or hypertension. The investigator of this study had a clear conceptual model that incorporated both physiologic and psychologic variables. Significant positive relationships between hardiness and psychosocial and physiologic adaptation were found *only* in the subsample (n = 20) with diabetes.

Evaluation of Nursing Interventions

Notably lacking in the decade of the 1980s was research designed to evaluate the effect of nursing interventions on individuals who have diabetes mellitus. Only two studies were found. In one, Massouh and associates (1989) examined the effect of a social learning intervention (that is, role-playing) on metabolic control in 39 adolescents with IDDM. Subjects were assigned randomly to participate in either a 40-minute role-modeling situation or a 40-minute session in which subjects were directed to review material previously presented to both groups. A single 40-minute role-modeling intervention was not sufficient to make any impact on metabolic control (glycosylated hemoglobin) measured three and one-half months later.

In another nursing intervention study, Jones (1990) evaluated the effectiveness of a 12-week self-study program, based on Kanfer's (1975) self-control theory, on adherence to following blood glucose self-monitoring goals. Thirty-four subjects with insulin-using diabetes were randomly assigned to either a self-study course or to a control group. The subjects completing the self-study program (n = 11) had significantly higher posttest scores than the control group (n = 14) on an investigator-developed tool to measure knowledge of self-control behavioral techniques. There was no difference in adherence to frequency of following blood glucose self-monitoring goals. A higher percentage of the control group (82%) reported following their blood glucose self-monitoring goals prior to the study than the treatment group (41%). A randomized design blocking on type of diabetes may have prevented this initial difference in subjects. The investigator also had problems with attrition and failed to evaluate if the treatment group actually used the self-control behavioral techniques.

Brown (1988) performed a meta-analysis of educational interventions on patient knowledge, self-care, and metabolic control conducted from 1954 to 1986. Forty-seven studies met the criteria for inclusion; that is, the investigators provided sufficient detail to estimate effect size and either included both a treatment and control group from the same setting or a one-group-pretest–posttest design. The weighted mean effect size for studies that included a control group was .40, whereas that for the one-group pretest–posttest design was .53. Together the weighted mean effect size was .33, adjusted for sample size and effect size variances, indicating that diabetes education for the average patient has a moderate positive effect. Brown (1990a) did a follow-up meta-analysis, including an additional 35 educational intervention studies published from 1986 to 1989, and found similar results. She noted that although there was a large increase in educational interventions from 1986 to 1989, very few of the published studies were nurse led ($n = 2$).

Brown (1990b) noted a number of methodologic considerations in reviewing the studies. A large percentage of the investigators did not report subject attrition: of those who did, many had high attrition rates. She also observed that diabetes educators develop new instruments to measure knowledge and self-care but seldom report reliability and validity.

SUMMARY AND DIRECTIONS FOR FUTURE RESEARCH

Most of the nursing diabetes research reviewed consisted of isolated studies that do not add to our understanding of how individuals with diabetes view their illness or whether nursing interventions are effective. Major methodologic problems existed in measurement and statistical application. Rigorous attention to reliability and validity to questionnaires and interviews was missing. A number of instruments measuring the same or similar concepts were newly developed by each succeeding investigator. Thus findings did not build on previous work.

A major methodologic problem in the studies reviewed was small samples. The need to take a multivariate approach in understanding compliance and diabetic control dictates larger samples. Use of multiple sites is the most obvious and direct way to increase subject pools. The competitive nature of health care delivery is often a barrier to collaboration across settings. Scientific review committees of major funding sources have the most power to change this by requiring multiple sites in grant applications.

Another methodologic problem in the studies reviewed was the lack of specification of types of diabetes. Nurse researchers often failed to report the criteria they used in classifying types of diabetes, which is a problem when attempting to compare results of studies by different researchers. Distinguishing between types of diabetes is directly related to decisions about treatment goals, which in turn, relate to how disease control is measured.

The research reviewed in this chapter could be placed into two groups. One group includes studies that predominately emerged from clinical problems such as patient reuse of insulin syringes. The other group of studies involves deductively applied models or theories to understand compliance, knowledge, and metabolic control in diabetes. These two groups of studies seem to represent the dichotomy often found between nurse researchers and nurse clinicians. This gap needs to be bridged to reach nurses' ultimate goal, the improvement of nursing care through incorporating research findings in clinical practice. Clinicians possess a wealth of knowledge about clinical problems, whereas nurse researchers have backgrounds in scientific methods and theory. Active collaboration between the two groups should lead to integration of theory, research, and practice.

An important area for research collaboration is measuring diabetic control. Clinicians and researchers together need to develop a multifactor measure that represents the complexity of the disease and differentiates between indicators of diabetic control for Type I and Type II diabetes. In addition, the cooperation of clinicians and nurse researchers could lead to frameworks that unite isolated clinical studies. A promising area for collaboration is the study of individuals adapting technology for daily self-care, and the effect that technology has on adaptation to diabetes and quality of life.

Several clinical issues germane to nursing care of individuals with diabetes have been addressed not at all or in only a limited manner. Among these relevant topics are prevention and early detection of NIDDM, prevention of complications such as neuropathies, integration of self-care technology, clarification of the relationship between stress and psychologic coping with disease control, description of the similarities and differences in populations with diabetes from diverse ethnic backgrounds, and identification of client and environmental characteristics that predict control. Instead of continuing to evaluate the effectiveness of isolated or generic diabetic teaching programs, nurse researchers should develop and evaluate models for client education during acute/critical health restoration as well as client education for maintaining disease control and preventing complications. In addition, the educational needs of individuals newly diagnosed with diabetes should be distinguished from individuals who have had diabetes for a number of years.

Means to promote and share nursing research in diabetes should be developed. Because there are few formal channels to share and disseminate information on instrument development, nurse researchers should establish informal networks among themselves and with other health professionals to share this information. Assessing reliability and validity of instruments in different settings by different investigators will enhance the development of instruments that have sound psychometric properties.

In summary, the paucity of nursing research in diabetes is disproportionate to the magnitude of the problems and the number of nurse clinicians providing care to individuals with diabetes. Research findings that are meaningful to practice will emerge only when nurse clinicians and researchers join together to unite theory, research, and practice.

REFERENCES

Ahern, J. A., Bates, S., & Tamborlane, W. V. (1988). Discrepancies between blood glucose and glycosylated hemoglobin in intensively treated diabetic patients. *The Diabetes Educator, 14*(1), 30–32.

Alogna, M. (1980). Perception of severity of disease and health locus of control in compliant and noncompliant diabetic patients. *Diabetes Care, 3,* 533–534.

Auerhahn, C., Bergman, M., Kumar, S. R., & Morgan, J. (1985). Reagent strip performance as evaluated by a meter. *The Diabetes Educator, 11*(4), 41–43.

Barr, B., Leichter, S. B., & Taylor, L. (1984). Bedside capillary glucose monitoring in the General Hospital. *Diabetes Care, 7,* 261–264.

Bennett, P. H. (1990). Epidemiology of diabetes mellitus. In H. Rifkin & D. Porte (Eds.), *Ellenberg and Rifkin's Diabetes Mellitus: Theory and practice* (pp. 357–377). New York: Elsevier.

Bloom-Cerkoney, K. A., & Hart, L. A. (1980). The relationship between the health belief model and compliance of persons with diabetes mellitus. *Diabetes Care, 3,* 594–598.

Brown, S. A. (1990a). Studies of educational interventions and outcomes in diabetic adults: A meta-analysis revisited. *Patient Education and Counseling, 16,* 189–215.

Brown, S. A. (1990b). Quality of reporting in diabetes patient education research: 1954–1986. *Research in Nursing and Health, 13,* 53–62.

Brown, S. A. (1988). Effects of educational interventions in diabetes care: A meta-analysis of findings. *Nursing Research, 37,* 223–230.

Burckhardt, C. S., Woods, S. L., Schultz, A. A., & Ziebarth, D. M. (1989). Quality of life of adults with chronic illness: A psychometric study. *Research in Nursing and Health, 12,* 347–354.

Coonrod, B. A., Ellis, D., Becker, D. J., Dorman, J. S., Drash, A. L., Kuller, L. H., & Orchard, T. J. (1989). Assessment of AlbuSure and its usefulness in identifying IDDM subjects at increased risk for developing clinical diabetic nephropathy. *Diabetes Care, 12,* 389–393.

Daschner, B. K. (1986). Problems perceived by adults in adhering to a prescribed diet. *The Diabetes Educator, 12*(2), 113–115.

D'Eramo-Melkus, G. A., & Demas, P. (1989). Patient perceptions of diabetes treatment goals. *The Diabetes Educator, 15*(5), 440–443.

Derogatis, L. R., & Melisaratos, N. (1983). The brief symptom inventory: An introductory report. *Psychological Medicine, 13*, 595–605.

Edelstein, J., & Linn, M. W. (1987). Locus of control and the control of diabetes. *The Diabetes Educator, 13*(1), 51–54.

Fairclough, P. K., Clements, R. S., Filer, D. V., & Bell, D. S. (1983). An evaluation of patient performance of and their satisfaction with various rapid blood glucose measurement systems. *Diabetes Care, 6*, 45–49.

Fox, M. A., Cassmeyer, V., Eaks, G. A., Hamera, E., O'Connell, K. A., & Knapp, T. (1984). Blood glucose self-monitoring usage and its influence on patients' perceptions of diabetes. *The Diabetes Educator, 1*(3), 27–31.

Freeman, C. (1986). The stability of chemstrip bG used in conjunction with AccuChek bG. *The Diabetes Educator, 12*(1), 28–29.

Frey, M. A., & Denyes, M. J. (1989). Health and illness self-care in adolescents with IDDM: A test of Orem's theory. *Advances in Nursing Science, 12*(1), 67–75.

Gabbay, K. H. (1976). Glycosylated hemoglobin and diabetic control. *New England Journal of Medicine, 295*, 443–444.

Germain, C. P., & Nemchik, R. M. (1988). Diabetes self-management and hospitalization. *Image: Journal of Nursing Scholarship, 20*, 74–78.

Gifford-Jorgensen, R. A., Borchert, J., Hassanein, R., Tilzer, L., Eaks, G. A., & Moore, W. A. (1986). Comparison of five glucose meters for self-monitoring of blood glucose by diabetic patients. *Diabetes Care, 9*, 70–76.

Giordano, B. P., Thrash, W., Hollenbaugh, L., Dube, W. P., Hodges, C., Swain, A., Banion, C. R., & Klingensmith, G. J. (1989). Performance of seven blood glucose testing systems at high altitude. *The Diabetes Educator, 15*(5), 444–448.

Given, W., Given, B. A., Gallin, R. S., & Condon, J. W. (1983). Development of scales to measure beliefs of diabetes patients. *Research in Nursing and Health, 6*, 127–141.

Grier, M. R., & Marquis, M. D. (1989). The presentation of scientific data in nursing research. In I. L. Abraham, D. M. Nadzam, J. J. Fitzpatrick, (Eds.), *Statistics and quantitative methods in nursing: Issues and strategies for research and education* (pp. 189–201). Philadelphia: Saunders.

Guinn, T. S., Bailey, G. J., & Mecklenburg, R. S. (1988). Factors related to discontinuation of continuous subcutaneous insulin-infusion therapy. *Diabetes Care, 11*, 46–51.

Hamera, E., Cassmeyer, V., O'Connell, K. A., Weldon, G. T., Knapp, T. M., & Kyner, J. L. (1988). Self-regulation in individuals with Type II diabetes. *Nursing Research, 37*, 363–367.

Havlin, C. E., & Cryer, P. E. (1987). Nocturnal hypoglycemia does not commonly result in major morning hyperglycemia in patients with diabetes mellitus. *Diabetes Care, 10*, 141–147.

Hite, M. A. (1982). Clinical estimation of the renal threshold for glucose in persons with diabetes mellitus. *Nursing Research, 31*, 153–158.

Jenkins, C. A., Powers, M. A., & Molitch, M. E. (1988). Comparison of ease of learning of four glucose meters. *The Diabetes Educator, 14*(4), 313–315.

Jones, P. M. (1990). Use of a course on self-control behavior techniques to increase adherence to prescribed frequency for self-monitoring blood glucose. *The Diabetes Educator, 16*(4), 296–303.

Kahn, L. B., Marshall, J. A., Baxter, J., Shetterly, S. M., & Hamman, R. F. (1990). Accuracy of reported family history of diabetes mellitus. *Diabetes Care, 13*(7), 796–798.

Kanfer, F. H. (1975). Self-management methods. In F. H. Kanfer & A. P. Goldstein (Eds.), *Helping people change* (pp. 309–55). New York: Pergamon Press.

Klosiewski, M. (1984). Hypoglycemia: What does the diabetic experience? *The Diabetes Educator, 10*(3), 18–21.

Lockwood, D., Frey, M. L., Gladish, N. A., & Hiss, R. G. (1986). The biggest problem in diabetes. *The Diabetes Educator, 12*(1), 30–33.

Lundman, B. (1988). Tedium among patients with insulin-dependent diabetes mellitus. *Journal of Advanced Nursing, 13,* 23–31.

Lundman, B., Asplund, K., & Norberg, A. (1988). Tedium among patients with insulin-dependent diabetes mellitus. *Journal of Advanced Nursing, 13,* 23–31.

Lundman, B., Asplund, K., & Norberg, A. (1990). Living with diabetes: Perceptions of well-being. *Research in Nursing and Health, 13,* 255–262.

Massouh, S. R., Steele, T. M. O., Alseth, E. R., & Diekmann, J. M. (1989). The effect of social learning intervention on metabolic control of insulin-dependent diabetes mellitus in adolescents. *The Diabetes Educator, 15*(6), 518–521.

Madsbad, S. (1990). Classification of diabetes in older adults. *Diabetes Care, 13*(suppl. 2), 93–96.

Meize-Grochowski, A. R. (1990). Health locus of control and glycosylated haemoglobin concentration of implantable insulin pump recipients in Austria. *Journal of Advanced Nursing, 15,* 804–807.

Nathan, P. M., Singer, D. E., Hurxthal, K., & Goodson, J. D. (1984). The clinical information value of the glycosylated hemoglobin assay. *New England Journal of Medicine, 310,* 341–346.

National Diabetes Data Group. (1985). *Diabetes in America* (NIH Publication No. 85-1468). Washington, DC: U.S. Department of Health and Human Services.

Nyhlin, K. T. (1990). Diabetic patients facing longterm complications: Coping with uncertainty. *Journal of Advanced Nursing, 15,* 1021–1029.

O'Connell, K. A., Hamera, E. K., Knapp, T. M., Cassmeyer, V. L., Eaks, G. A., & Fox, M. A. (1984). Symptom and self-regulation in type II diabetes. *Advances in Nursing Science, 6*(3), 19–28.

O'Connell, K. A., Hamera, E. K., Schorfheide, A., & Guthrie, D. (1990). Symptom beliefs and actual blood glucose in type II diabetes. *Research in Nursing and Health, 13,* 145–151.

Orem, D. E. (1991). Nursing: Concepts of Practice (4th ed.). St. Louis, MO: Mosby.

Pieper, B. A., Kushion, W., & Gaida, S. (1990). The relationship between a couple's marital adjustment and beliefs about diabetes mellitus. *The Diabetes Educator, 16*(2), 108–112.

Pollock, S. E. (1989). Adaptive responses to diabetes mellitus. *Western Journal of Nursing Research, 11,* 265–280.

Pollock, S. E. (1986). Human responses to chronic illness: Physiologic and psychosocial adaptation. *Nursing Research, 35,* 90–95.

Poteet, G. W., Reinert, B., & Ptak, H. E. (1987). Outcome of multiple usage of disposable syringes in the insulin-requiring diabetic. *Nursing Research, 36,* 350–352.

Primomo, J., Yates, B. C., & Woods, N. F. (1990). Social support for women during chronic illness: The relationship among sources and types to adjustment. *Research in Nursing and Health, 13,* 153–161.

Saucier, C. P. (1984). Improvement in long-term control of children performing blood glucose self-monitoring. *The Diabetes Educator, 10*(3), 33–35.

Schlenk, E. A., & Hart, L. K. (1984). Relationship between health locus of control, health value, and social support and compliance of persons with diabetes mellitus. *Diabetes Care, 7,* 566–574.

Teza, S. L., Davis, W. K., & Hiss, R. G. (1988). Patient knowledge compared with national guidelines for diabetes care. *The Diabetes Educator, 14*(3), 207–211.

Turner, J. G., & Lancaster, J. (1984). Multiple use of disposable syringe units by insulin-dependent diabetics. *The Diabetes Educator, 10*(3), 38–41.

Wakefield, B., Wilberding, J. Z., Wakefield, S. D., Booth, B. M., & Buckwalter, K. C. (1989). Does contamination affect the reliability and validity of bisected chemstrip bGs? *Western Journal of Nursing Research, 11,* 328–333.

Watkins, J. D., Roberts, D. E., Williams, T. F., Martin, D. A., & Coyle, V. (1967a). Observation of medication errors made by diabetic patients in the home. *Diabetes, 16,* 882–885.

Watkins, J. D., Williams, T. F., Martin, D. A., Hogan, M. D., & Anderson, E. (1967b). A study of diabetic patients at home. *American Journal of Public Health, 57,* 452–459.

Wierenga, M. E., Browning, J. M., & Mahn, J. L. (1990). A descriptive study of how clients make life-style changes. *The Diabetes Educator, 16*(6), 469–473.

Wikblad, K. F., Wibell, L. B., & Montin, K. R. (1990). The patient's experience of diabetes and its treatment: Construction of an attitude scale by a semantic differential technique. *Journal of Advanced Nursing, 15,* 1083–1091.

Williams, T. F., Anderson, E., Watkins, J. D., & Coyle, V. (1967). Dietary errors made at home by patients with diabetes. *Journal of the American Dietetic Association, 51,* 19–25.

Williams, T. F., Martin, D. A., Hogan, M. D., Watkins, J. D., & Ellis, E. V. (1967). The clinical picture of diabetic control studied in four settings. *American Journal of Public Health, 57,* 441–451.

Chapter 4

Battered Women and Their Children

JACQUELYN C. CAMPBELL
COLLEGE OF NURSING
WAYNE STATE UNIVERSITY

BARBARA PARKER
SCHOOL OF NURSING
UNIVERSITY OF MARYLAND

CONTENTS

The battering of women has been recognized as a serious social and health problem. Nursing research has added a unique perspective to knowledge development in the field of woman abuse. Literature in other disciplines has been concentrated on either causation or psychologic problems from abuse. Nurse researchers have been more concerned with responses to and characteristics of woman abuse. In addition to the emotional and behavioral reactions usually studied, nurse investigators have included physical injury and physical responses in their research on woman abuse.

This review is limited to data-based inquiries related to physical, sexual, or emotional abuse of female partners and the effects of that abuse on their children. Studies published in nursing journals or studies in violence-related interdisciplinary journals conducted by authors who identify themselves as nurses were included. A *MEDLINE* search from 1970 to 1990 was conducted and the *Cumulative Index to Nursing and Allied Health Literature* was searched for the same years. A hand search was conducted of the five interdisciplinary journals specific to violence for their entire years of publication (*Victimology, Journal of Interpersonal Violence, Journal of Family Violence, Response to the Victimization of Women and Children,* and *Violence and Victims*). Reference lists of the articles found also were used to identify additional references. Finally, nurse researchers who listed wife abuse as a topic of research in the *Sigma Theta Tau Directory of Nurse Researchers* (2nd edition, 1987) were sent letters requesting their published research.

The review begins with a brief introduction to the state of the science in battering research, including the methodologic limitations in the field in general. This is followed by a description of the general state of the science in nursing research on the subject. The specific review is divided into the following categories: women's responses to battering (physical, emotional, behavioral), battering during pregnancy, children of battered women, homicide in battering relationships, wife rape, battered women in the health care setting, and nurses' attitudes toward battered women.

OVERVIEW OF RESEARCH ON BATTERING

The earliest studies of wife abuse were psychiatric case studies interpreting the behavior of both the batterer and his wife as evidence of psychiatric pathology, with an assumption of female masochism (e.g., Snell, Rosenwald, & Robey, 1964). Partly in response to the feminist movement in the late 1960s, attempts were made to document battering as a widespread problem starting with O'Brien's (1971) landmark review of divorce cases (16.7% spontaneous mention of abuse) and culminating with the 1980 and 1990 national random surveys of family violence (Straus & Gelles, 1990; Straus, Gelles, & Steinmetz, 1980). A baseline prevalence of one in four couples ever using violence and four of every 100 wives seriously abused was established from these surveys. This rate did not change significantly over the 10 years.

Sociologic research has moved from descriptive studies to a concentration on causation, with the major theoretical frameworks of exchange, feminism, social learning, stress, and systems all receiving some research support (Van Hasselt, Morrison, Bellack, & Hersen, 1988). Psychologic studies of both batterers and battered women have established some common characteristics of abusive men as more likely to have been exposed to violence as a child, and to have chronic alcohol problems and problems related to self-perceived inability to fulfill traditional male roles and/or needs for control without mechanisms to exert power (Tolman & Bennett, 1990). Low socioeconomic status was identified as the only consistent risk for woman abuse, whereas depression and low self-esteem of abused women have been identified as responses to the abuse rather than risk factors for abuse (Hotaling & Sugarman, 1990).

The limitations in the entire field of research on battering have included operational discrepancies, both measurement and definitional. Over time it has been recognized that abuse of female partners is a singular phenomenon that includes sexual, emotional, and physical abuse. The dynamics are similar, whether or not the partners are legally married. However, there are still separate bodies of literature, dividing the field into wife abuse, marital rape, dating violence, and date rape. There is also controversy over whether the phenomenon of abuse should be regarded as "conjugal" or "domestic" violence and considered as part of family violence or woman abuse and viewed as part of violence against women (see Straus & Gelles, 1990, and Yllo & Bograd, 1988, for both sides of this debate). However, in this review battering is defined as repeated, deliberate physical (including sexual) assault within a context of coercive control. This kind of violence is directed primarily toward female partners in intimate relationships. Thus, gender specific terminology will be used. In this chapter *abuse* is used as a term encompassing emotional, sexual, and material degradation and threats as well as physical and sexual assault.

An extension of the definitional controversy is the issue of measurement, since the most widely used instrument for domestic violence is the Conflict Tactics Scale (CTS) (Straus & Gelles, 1990). This instrument measures the frequency and severity of tactics used in disagreements. Because it omits the extent of injury, self-defense, sexual assault, and emotional degradation, the female partner's behavior is scored as being as violent as the male's. Therefore, the scale has been challenged as invalid for measuring battering as defined in this review (Saunders, 1986).

Other limitations of the research have been a slowness in inclusion of cultural influences, limited theory testing research, few experimental studies to evaluate interventions, and overuse of women and children in shelters or treatment agencies. In addition, woman abuse research has been criticized for its dependence on reports of the survivor without validating the occurrence of the violent behavior with the aggressor, although Uphold and Strickland

(1989) note that the use of one informant in family study may be preferable. Public health and medicine have been slow to recognize the health implications of battering and are only beginning to conduct research from their disciplinary perspectives. There is also an ongoing controversy between traditional social scientists and those who call for an "activist research" approach, aligning themselves with the grassroots battered women's movement, feminist theory, and critical theory (Dobash & Dobash, 1988). These researchers and activists want to make sure that the primary agenda for future research on battering is to empower the women and children involved and to put the onus of responsibility on the social system to change, rather than the individual women (Parker, 1988).

Nurses who conduct research on battering have, for the most part, worked closely with abused women in health care settings and/or in shelters, with their inquiry growing out of clinical concerns. Their research is therefore congruent with the activist research agenda. An example of research on battering during pregnancy using feminist principles to empower clinical nurse data collectors has recently been described (Parker & McFarlane, 1991). There also is considerable concern among nursing researchers for the safety of abused women used as research subjects (Parker et al., 1990). Nurse researchers' knowledge of and ability to influence the health care system in combination with a women's health orientation and social responsibility stance affords nurse researchers a unique and crucial part in that agenda (Campbell, 1988).

Nursing research to date has ranged from descriptive small-sample studies to model testing, experimental designs, and sophisticated qualitative analytic approaches. The studies emcompassed incidence reports in specific populations, identification of causative factors, and responses to victimization. There have been no nursing theory testing studies and limited nursing theory application work in the area, the most notable being a clinically based application of Roy's Adaptation Model (Limandri, 1986), a theory extension study of dependent care in battered women and their children (Humphreys, 1991), a homicide prediction instrument framed within Orem's theory of self-care (Campbell, 1986a), and a case study applying Parse's theory to a couple in an abusive relationship (Butler & Snodgrass, 1991).

In terms of sampling, some of the early researchers used very small clinical samples and several nurse investigators have used shelter populations to describe phenomena such as ethnic differences with survivors (Torres, 1987, 1991), appropriate social support (Henderson, 1989), and use of support groups (Campbell, 1986b; Trimpey, 1989). There have been a number of studies that have extended the sites to nontraditional populations such as legal aide bureaus (Parker & Schumacher, 1977), community settings (Campbell, 1989a; Landenburger, 1989; Ulrich, 1991), primary care settings including women's health centers (Bullock, McFarlane, Bateman, & Miller, 1989), prenatal clinics (Helton, McFarlane, & Anderson, 1987; McFarlane et al., in press), and postpartum units (Bullock & McFarlane, 1989) as well as public institutions, such as schools (Bullock & McFarlane, 1989) and universities (King & Ryan, 1989). These diverse settings have added depth and richness to research on women abuse that is not always found in research from other disciplines.

Nursing research has been facilitated by a recent article by the Nursing Research Consortium on Violence and Abuse delineating a safety protocol for research on abuse of women (Parker et al., 1990). This article, included as a protocol in applications to Institutional Review Boards (IRBs), has helped researchers in obtaining IRB approval from committees who are appropriately concerned with issues of the woman's safety.

WOMEN'S RESPONSES TO BATTERING

Physical Response

How women respond to repeated acts of violence in an intimate partner relationship can be conceptually divided into physical, psychologic, and behavioral responses. Physical responses have been measured in two nursing studies. In a descriptive study of 130 Canadian women in a shelter, Kerouac and her associates (Kerouac, Taggart, Lescop, & Fortin, 1986) reported that 20.7% of the sample stated they were bothered by sleep disturbances and disturbing physical sensations, 20% by asthma, 11.6% by allergies, and 7.7% by arthritis. However, just over half the women perceived their health status as excellent or good. Although in that study researchers did not use a comparison group for physical responses, Campbell's (1989a) comparison group study found a group of battered women ($N = 97$) to have significantly more troublesome stress-related symptoms than a group of other women ($N = 96$) also having significant problems in an intimate relationship. The sample, both economically and ethnically diverse, was recruited from the community using newspaper advertisement. Physical symptoms was one of two significant differences between the groups. The other difference was that the abused women had thought of or tried significantly *more* solutions to the relationship problems.

Psychologic Responses

In terms of emotional responses, the two groups of women in the Campbell (1989a) research were not significantly different on mean levels of depression or self-esteem, but there were proportionately more battered women who were seriously depressed. Both groups were significantly below the norms on the Tennessee Self Concept Scale (Fitts, 1972). Mahon (1981) also found significantly lower scores on ego strength using the *Cattell 16PF Questionnaire* (Cattell, 1969) but significantly greater self-sufficiency. However, the small sample ($N = 11$) limited the usefulness of Mahon's findings. Trimpey's (1989) sample of 36 women from a shelter support group also showed significantly lowered self-esteem and increased anxiety using other normed instruments. Unfortunately, in the discussion of findings, Trimpey did not address the possible influence of demographic differences (i.e., 62% of the abused women reported an income of $10,000 or less and 67% of the subjects were currently residing in a shelter for battered women) between the abused women and the instrument norm groups of working and college women and male patients with anxiety and depressive reactions. Trimpey did note the possible influence of the instruments being administered during the often stressful first visit to a support group.

Thus, there is support in nursing research for problems with self-esteem in battered women as well as some indication of anxiety and depression. However, these emotional problems, which can also occur without physical violence, can be viewed as part of a response to the actual or threatened loss of the woman's most important attachment relationship. Campbell's (1989a) quantitative comparison of grief and learned helplessness models found equal support for the grief framework and the more pathologically oriented learned helplessness response. Rosenbaum (1988) has argued that maritally discordant couples are a more appropriate comparison group for abusive couples than "normal" couples if the factors specific to violence are to be identified.

Nurse investigators have also suggested that abused women display emotional strength in some areas. This has been elucidated in qualitative studies by Landenburger (1988, 1989), Hoff (1990), and Ulrich (1991).

Landenburger (1988, 1989) used a triangulation design to identify a process of entrapment in and recovery from an abusive relationship. Thirty women from both shelters and the community were interviewed using an ethnographic interview schedule, phenomenology principles, and both domain and comparative analytic strategies. This work helped to illuminate the process that women go through in the course of an abusive relationship and to explain why women respond differently, both to the violence and to people trying to provide help, at different points in time. Landenburger identified stages of binding, which included aspects of self-blame, covering up the abuse, and "shrinking of the self"; disengaging, a period of help seeking; and recovering, wherein she completes grief work, tries to find meaning in her experience, and works at the pragmatics of survival.

Ulrich's sample of 51 formerly abused women also tended to describe leaving as a process prompted by multiple and varied reasons. Using content analysis with a careful reliability check, Ulrich categorized women's reasons for leaving an abusive relationship into the two major themes of safety, including personal safety and emotional safety of the children, and personal growth, reaching a new understanding or concern for one's own potential. Dependency on an outside entity was a third theme but listed by only three women.

Hoff's (1990) ethnographic study of nine battered women and 131 social network members over a 2-year period also added insight to the process, which Hoff labeled as going from victim to survivor. In this work, Hoff elucidated the complex interactional process among personal, cultural, and political-economic factors that contribute to women feeling entrapped in a violent relationship. Furthermore, Hoff demonstrated how the women in her study were successful crisis managers in their day-to-day lives, but that the social system continually defined the larger problem of battering as a personal one, thus contributing to the women's attempts to solve the problem of being battered on a private level (Hoff, 1990; Landenburger, 1984, 1989; Ulrich, 1991). All of these studies were of predominantly white women and need to be replicated with culturally diverse samples.

Behavioral Responses

The majority of research on battered women has been on how women behave when confronted with battering from a male partner. The work of Torres (1987, 1991) has provided a needed cultural comparison of some of the responses of women to abuse. She found 25 Hispanic-American battered women to have experienced similar frequency and severity of violence as 25 Anglo-American women in shelters. However, the Hispanic-American women were more tolerant of the abuse. In addition, concern for the children was the most important issue for 40% of the Hispanic women in their decisions to leave or stay with the child's father, while it was most important for 20% of the Anglo women. Lichtenstein (1981) found a similar percentage of primarily Anglo-American women (N = 30) citing their children's welfare as a primary reason for staying and/or returning. The importance of cultural considerations also was demonstrated in the Torres (1987, 1991) analysis. Torres found the tendency of the Hispanic-American women to stay in the relationship longer related to pressure from extended family and/or threats to family members, whereas Anglo-American women in both samples were more influenced by lack of resources. Hoff (1990) found the families of her primarily Anglo-American sample to be supportive of the women. Poverty was important but not the primary factor in decisions to stay in the relationship.

Parker and Schumacher (1977) also have provided insights into the process of leaving or remaining in a battering relationship. The Parker and

Schumacher work is considered classic in the field of woman abuse. The work is consistently cited by researchers in all disciplines as one of the first controlled wife abuse investigations. In the article, the investigators also introduced the term *battered wife syndrome* to describe a symptom complex occurring when a wife received deliberate, severe, and repeated (more than three times) demonstrable injury from her husband. This early definition was later extended by Walker (1979) and others to apply to unmarried couples but unfortunately was expanded to include an assumption of psychologic deficits ascribed to all battered women. Parker and Schumacher (1977) were careful to identify a separate group of abused women (violence syndrome averters) who were able to decrease the violence either by leaving or by getting help. These women were more likely to have never observed their mothers beaten by their fathers.

In three separate studies nurses have examined the influence of social support on the behavioral responses to abuse. Hoff (1988, 1990), using feminist ethnographic methodology, documented a different picture than commonly assumed for battered women in terms of informal support. Most women reported at least some family or friends who were supportive. The women reported that they did not feel isolated, although their batterer often tried to impose isolation. However, Hoff (1990) found her sample's natural network to be insufficient and the formal system unresponsive.

Henderson (1989) and Campbell (1986b) used qualitative data to examine support provided by shelters. Henderson interviewed eight women to identify four stages of need for support in a shelter: (a) reassurance, when the woman gathered information to make sense of the past; (b) analysis, after which they were able to put the past into perspective; (c) reciprocity, when the women gave back to newly arriving residents, a stage as important to the giver of support as to those receiving; and (d) independence, the period of adjustment accompanied by feelings of self-growth, which started in the shelter but was mainly concluded after leaving the shelter. Both Campbell (1986b) and Henderson (1989) describe patterns or stages in the immediate shelter recovery period. These included decision making regarding the relationship, mutual sharing and support, and reciprocity between the women as they supported each other in recovery. The description of these stages generally supported the findings by Landenburger (1988, 1989) of her stages of disengagement and recovery.

The themes identified by Campbell (1986b) in her analysis of shelter support group meetings provided further contextual documentation of abused women's active participation in mutual affirmation support in the process of recovering. Women's search for meaning in the abusive relationship also was a major theme. All five qualitative studies (Campbell, 1986; Henderson, 1987; Hoff, 1990; Landenburger, 1989; Ulrich, 1991) were strengthened by using battered women to validate the findings; however, Campbell's (1986b) analysis had no reliability (verifiability) assessment in contrast to the other studies.

BATTERING DURING PREGNANCY

The work of Helton, McFarlane, and Anderson (1987) established a baseline prevalence of approximately 8% to 9% of pregnant women who were physically abused during the current pregnancy. This is consistent with the findings of others (e.g., Campbell, Poland, Waller, & Ager, in press; Hillard, 1985). An additional 15% to 21% of women were beaten during the year prior to the pregnancy, making them highly at risk for further abuse as well as subject to the atmosphere of threat and coercive control that accompanies physical violence (Helton, 1986; Helton et al., 1987). Important additional findings were that demographic variables, including ethnicity in a balanced sample of 290 African-American, Mexican-American, and European-American women, did not predict abuse during pregnancy, whereas physical violence before pregnancy did. In a postpartum extension of the research, Bullock and McFarlane (1989) corroborated the prevalence and demographic findings of prenatal abuse documented in the earlier work. They also found a significant correlation between prenatal battering and birthweight, even controlling for race, smoking, alcohol consumption, prenatal care, abortions, and other maternal complications in a sample of 589 women. Other detrimental infant outcomes, such as miscarriages from abuse (Brendtro & Bowker, 1989), have been suggested in retrospective studies but not yet established in cohort designs.

McFarlane and colleagues (in press), in a prospective prenatal study of over 700 Hispanic-American, African-American, and Anglo-American patients, found the rate of abuse was 25% in the year preceding pregnancy and 16% during pregnancy. This study also documented a significant relationship between experiencing abuse and entering prenatal care later in the pregnancy.

Lia-Hoagberg, Knoll, Swaney, Carlson, and Mullett (1988) also studied abuse in pregnancy as one of 40 psychosocial factors in their retrospective comparative study of 65 women who delivered low-birth-weight infants to 65 mothers of normal-birth-weight infants. The authors found an incidence of physical abuse of 12% in low-birth-weight mothers compared to 10.8% in normal-birth-weight mothers. The only statistically significant differences between the two groups were hospitalizations and the use of street drugs during pregnancy. One potential problem with the design of this study, however, was its reliance on medical records to document both the use of street drugs and the presence of physical or emotional abuse. Both problems are more likely to be uncovered when specifically assessed by trained observers (Parker & McFarlane, 1991).

In a similar finding related to the use of street drugs, Campbell and her associates (in press) found that violence during pregnancy was positively related to drug abuse during pregnancy in a postpartum sample of 900 poor African-American women in an urban area. The investigators found that a decrease in adequate prenatal care and an increase in alcohol abuse were associated with physical violence from a male partner. Similar to nonpregnant women, anxiety and depression were associated with abuse in this postpartum sample. In spite of the large sample, this study was limited by the battering inquiry being a secondary issue and therefore neither operationalized adequately nor appropriate for multivariate analysis.

CHILDREN OF ABUSED WOMEN

In a few studies nurses have examined the effects of growing up in a violent home on the children of abused women. Westra and Martin (1981) used physical measurements, a neurologic examination, developmental assessments, and interviews to assess 20 children (average age of 5) in a shelter for battered women. The children scored significantly lower on cognitive and motor tasks and behaved more aggressively than children from nonviolent homes, but the physical examinations were within normal limits. Kerouac and her associates (1986) reported that battered women perceived the majority of their children to enjoy normal health; however, their children actually had more diagnosable health problems than province (Quebec) norms. The 130 children (mean age of 6.5 years) also exhibited learning and behavioral problems. Neither of the two research teams (Kerouac et al., 1986; Westra & Martin, 1981) compared the prevalence of social and psychologic problems of the children with normative groups nor did they take into account the immediate stress of shelter living on children's performance and behavior.

Additionally, in other studies nurses have examined the influence in adulthood of growing up in a violent home. For example, Stuart, Laraia, Ballenger, and Lydiard (1990) found a history of sexual mistreatment in 50% of women with bulimia and 40% of women with depression, whereas 28% of the normal controls identified a history of sexual mistreatment. In addition, bulimics were raised in households with significantly more tension, threats, and physically coercive behavior than controls, although the use of physical violence was not significant.

HOMICIDE

Lichtenstein (1981) found that one of the influences on women's behavioral responses to battering is realistic fear of homicide. Campbell's (1981, in press) feminist framework using historical and epidemiologic exploration of homicide of women in Dayton, Ohio, between 1975 and 1979, was the beginning of her program of research with battered women. Fifty-seven percent of those homicides that involved adult women were between intimate partners, that is, current or estranged husband and wife or boyfriend and girlfriend. In at least two-thirds of all the cases, the woman had been battered before the homicide. When a woman killed her current or ex-partner, the man was the first to use violence in the altercation in 80% of the cases. The cases of men killing their ex-wives and ex-girlfriends or killing their wives when the wives said they wanted a divorce verified battered women's fears that their husbands would kill them if they left.

Based on the Ohio study and literature review of other retrospective homicide studies, a clinical assessment instrument, the Danger Assessment, for helping battered women determine their relative risk of homicide in the relationship was developed. The original instrument development work indicated initial support for internal consistency reliability and concurrent construct validity. Stuart and Campbell (1989) found additional reliability and validity support for the instrument in a small sample ($N = 30$) and the indication that an additional item on suicide threats by the male partner should be added. Foster, Veale, and Fogle (1989) added important information about women who killed their abuser from a very small ($N = 12$) retrospective study of those incarcerated. The incarcerated women reported emotional abuse and isolation as important precipitating factors, but they did not perceive escalation of violence and sexual abuse as risk factors for murdering abusive husbands. The Danger Assessment instrument needs considerable work, especially predictive validity assessment, before it can be considered an empirically useful instrument. However, the testing of the instrument to date supports clinical relevance and continuation in research development.

SEXUAL ABUSE

Several researchers (e.g., Brendtro & Bowker, 1989; Campbell, 1989b; Russell, 1982) have found that at least 45% of all battered women also were sexually assaulted. This sexual assault fits the criminal definitions for rape and often was referred to as marital rape in the literature. However, because these assaults are usually repeated in the context of a battering relationship, the term *sexual abuse* may be more accurate. In a sample of 97 battered women, Campbell (1989a) found that self-esteem and body image scores were significantly correlated with sexual abuse, even when controlling for frequency and severity of physical violence. Sexual abuse also was correlated with more frequent and severe physical violence in the relationship. In a sample of women in shelters ($N = 120$), Campbell and Alford (1989) reported women's perceptions of serious physical consequences, including vaginal and anal infections, tearing, and chronic pain, from sexual abuse.

Weingourt (1990) studied women being treated for primary depression or anxiety ($N = 53$). She found that the majority (62%) had been raped by their husband and approximately half of those were battered as well as raped. Only two women had been forced into sex by their husband on a single occasion; the rest had repeatedly been sexually abused. A history of child sexual abuse was significantly related to wife rape in this sample. This study is particularly important in documenting the importance of sexual abuse as a problem separate from physical assault. Both the Weingourt (1990) study and the Campbell and Alford (1989) research were limited by a lack of complete description of the sample demographics and descriptive analytic procedures.

BATTERED WOMEN IN THE HEALTH CARE SYSTEM

Several research efforts have been aimed at identification of battered women in the health care system, in terms of both establishing prevalence in various populations and determining how best to assess for battering. There also have been investigations of attitudes of health care professionals conducted.

Emergency Departments

In three studies data were elicited about emergency department (ED) visits from battered women. Drake's (1982) study was a small ($N = 12$) retrospective pilot, Goldberg and Tomlanovich (1984) surveyed 492 urban emergency room patients while waiting for care, and Stark et al. (1981) reviewed 481 ED patient charts. All three samples were primarily African-American and European-American, ranging in proportion from approximately 50:50 to 30:70. The cumulative data from the different methods and different geographic locations indicated that battered women were a significant proportion (at least 10% to 22% and probably as much as 25%) of women in emergency settings, were sustaining significant injuries from the beatings and wanted to receive services specific to abuse from health care professionals. However, only 2%

to 8% were identified as abused on their records and they did not receive as much or as useful assistance as they wanted.

Stark et al. (1981) documented significantly increased prescriptions of minor tranquilizers and pain medications of abused women than for other women in the emergency department whereas Goldberg and Tomlanovich (1984) did not, possibly because they did not control for gender in that analysis. Stark and his colleagues interpreted the increased prescriptions as evidence of the health care system's perpetuation of abuse, as these medications might serve to blunt the woman's motivations to end the relationship. However, Goldberg and Tomlanovich (1984) found an increased prevalence of chronic pain in spouse abuse victims. Thus, pain medication may be the appropriate intervention. A useful, as yet unexplored topic would be to compare tranquilizer prescriptions in abused versus not abused women, controlling for severity of anxiety complaints.

The Goldberg and Tomlanovich (1984) finding that chronic pain was the most frequent complaint in their sample of battered women, and the Stark et al. (1981) reporting of a pattern of proximal rather than distal injuries have been particularly useful in subsequent identification of abused women in emergency departments and the development of protocols. Drake's (1982) research report used extensive quotes giving compelling evidence of the lack of sensitive care from the health care system and the kinds of barriers to care these women perceived. For instance, women discussed being prevented from seeking health care by their male partner or not being sure if he would be notified if she went without him. Researchers from other disciplines (e.g., Kurz, 1987) also have documented the problems battered women encounter in the health care setting. Research findings have been instrumental in changing the approach of many emergency departments to wife abuse and are the basis of most emergency protocols in use today. One myth, that abused women hide their battering from health care professionals and/or find questioning about abuse intrusive, was effectively dispelled by Drake's work.

Tilden and Shepherd (1987), using a carefully designed time-series quasi experiment, demonstrated a significant increase in nurses' documentation of battering after staff training and implementation of an abuse victim protocol. However, the increase from 9.72% recorded identification to 22.97%, although significant, was not to an optimal level.

The findings of Brendtro and Bowker (1989) supported the lack of identification and useful interventions by health care professionals. The least effective formal source of help identified in their survey was "health care personnel." Only 31% of the women gave a very or somewhat effective rating to health care personnel compared to 56% (the largest percentage) giving that rating to battered women's shelters. One problem with the Brendtro and Bowker study was its failure to differentiate types of health care personnel.

Other Health Care Settings

Bullock et al., (1989) reviewed records (N = 793) in a Planned Parenthood clinic where intake forms included four questions about violence. An 8.2% prevalence rate was found, indicating a significant intervention opportunity and an easy method of assessment for abuse. All staff were trained in the dynamics and assessment of abuse; the nurse practitioners were trained in interventions for those battered. Battered women in the sample also were found to have significantly more recent life changes as well as parenting, legal, and emotional problems.

ATTITUDE STUDIES

Shipley and Sylvester (1982) and Rose and Saunders (1986) compared nurses with other health care professionals. In the comparisons, both nurses and physicians believed some myths about battered women, including that women are at least somewhat responsible for their victimization. Although the Rose and Saunders (1986) study seemed to indicate that nurses were less victim blaming and more sympathetic than physicians, gender rather than profession was the differentiating factor. However, backgrounds including intensive training (Rose & Saunders, 1986) and increased clinical contact with victims (Shipley & Sylvester, 1982) increased sensitivity in all groups. The King and Ryan (1989) work was important in documenting the tendency of clinical nurses to use a paternalistic rather than empowering model of helping with abused women. Specific training on abuse, including affective domain work, intervention philosophies, and clinical experience is needed in basic and continuing nursing education.

SUMMARY AND FUTURE DIRECTIONS

Nurse researchers have developed beginning programs of research in women abuse. Some of the studies reviewed have very small samples and/or unsophisticated methodologies; however, the findings from those studies in many cases are supported by more advanced research, both inside and outside nursing. Nursing is approaching a point where the database can be generalized or at least used as a starting point for nursing interventions in multiple settings.

The findings accumulated thus far include that at least 8% of women in prenatal and primary care settings are abused by a male partner and approximately 20% of women in emergency departments have a history of abuse.

Obviously, this prevalence data coupled with consistent findings of significant health problems, lack of documentation, and abused women's perceptions of poor care by health care professionals indicates a need for continuing and basic education in nursing. Tilden and Shepherd (1987) have provided evidence of the effectiveness of a training program for emergency nursing, but further studies like theirs are needed in other arenas.

Nurse researchers have also documented a consistent finding of problems in self-esteem in battered women, perhaps especially in those also sexually abused. In addition to other findings of emotional problems, nurse researchers have identified significant strengths of battered women, indications of normal processes of grieving and recovering, and cultural and social support influences on responses to battering. These findings taken cumulatively are beginning to indicate data-based nursing interventions that will in many cases duplicate the clinical suggestions already in the literature. The emphasis on strengths, rather than pathology, and the implications for interventions that empower rather than patronize are important advances. However, clinical trials testing nursing interventions have yet to be published, and this is a serious weakness in nursing research to date. Other gaps include systematic inquiry into the kinds of health problems battered women may demonstrate and whether or not the batterer prevents appropriate use of health care services. Theory development and extension and/or further testing of theory applications are essential for the knowledge base to expand nursing science.

REFERENCES

Brendtro, M., & Bowker, H. L. (1989). Battered women: How can nurses help. *Issues in Mental Health Nursing, 10,* 169–180.

Bullock, L., & McFarlane, J. (1989). Higher prevalence of low birthweight infants born to battered women. *American Journal of Nursing, 89,* 1153–1155.

Bullock, L., McFarlane, J., Bateman, L., & Miller, V. (1989). Characteristics of battered women in a primary care setting. *Nurse Practitioner, 14*(6), 47–51.

Butler, M., & Snodgrass, F. (1991). Beyond abuse: Parse's Theory in action. *Nursing Science Quarterly, 4*(2), 76–82.

Campbell, J. C. (1981). Misogyny and homicide of women. *Advances in Nursing Science, 3*(2), 67–85.

Campbell, J. C. (1986a). Nursing assessment of homicide with battered women. *Advances in Nursing Science, 8*(4), 36–51.

Campbell, J. C. (1986b). A survivor group for battered women. *Advances in Nursing Science, 8*(2), 13–20.

Campbell, J. C. (1988). Nursing and battered women. *Response, 11*(2), 21–23.

Campbell, J. C. (1989a). A test of two explanatory models of women's responses to battering. *Nursing Research, 38,* 18–24.

Campbell, J. C. (1989b). Women's responses to sexual abuse in intimate relationships. *Women's Health Care International, 8,* 335–347.

Campbell, J. C. (in press). "If I can't have you, no one can": Issues of power and control in homicide of female partners. In J. Randford & D. Russell (Eds.), *Femicide: The politics of woman killing*. Boston, MA: Twayne Publishers.

Campbell, J. C., & Alford, P. (1989). Women's response to sexual abuse in intimate relationships. *American Journal of Nursing, 84,* 946–949.

Campbell, J. C., Poland, M. L., Waller, J. B., & Ager, J. A. (In press). Correlates of battering during pregnancy. *Research in Nursing and Health.*

Cattell, R. B. (1969). *16 PF Questionnaire*. Champaign, IL: Institute for Personality and Ability Testing.

Dobash, R. E., & Dobash, R. (1988). Research as social action: The struggle for battered women. In K. Yllo & M. Bograd (Eds.), *Feminist perspectives on wife abuse* (pp. 51–74). Beverly Hills, CA: Sage.

Drake, V. K. (1982). Battered women: A health care problem in disguise. *Image: Journal of Nursing Scholarship, 14,* 40–47.

Fitts, W. H. (1972). *The self concept and behavior: Overview and supplement.* Nashville, TN: Dade Wallace Center Services.

Foster, L. A., Veale, C. M., & Foge, C. I. (1989). Factors present when battered women kill. *Issues in Mental Health Nursing, 10,* 273–284.

Goldberg, W. G., & Tomlanovich, M. C. (1984). Domestic violence victims in the emergency department. *Journal of the American Medical Association, 251,* 3259–3264.

Helton, A. (1986). The pregnant battered woman. *Response, 19,* 22–23.

Helton, A. S., McFarlane, J., & Anderson, E. T. (1987). Battered and pregnant: A prevalence study. *American Journal of Public Health, 77,* 1337–1339.

Henderson, D. A. (1989). Use of social support in a transition house for abused women. *Health Care for Women International, 10*(1), 61–73.

Hillard, P. J. (1985). Physical abuse in pregnancy. *Obstetrics and Gynecology, 66,* 185–190.

Hoff, L. A. (1988). Collaborative feminist research and the myth of objectivity. In K. Yllo & M. Bograd (Eds.) *Feminist perspectives on wife abuse* (pp. 269–281). Newbury Park, CA: Sage.

Hoff, L. A. (1990). *Battered women as survivors*. London: Routledge.

Hotaling, G. T., & Sugarman, D. B. (1990). A risk marker analysis of assaulted wives. *Journal of Family Violence, 5,* 1–14.

Humphreys, J. C. (1991). Children of battered women: Worries about their mother. *Pediatric Nursing, 17,* 342–345.

Kerouac, S., Taggart, M. E., Lescop, J., & Fortin, M. F. (1986). Dimensions of health in violent families. *Health Care for Women International, 7,* 413–426.

King, M. C., & Ryan, J. (1989). Abused women: Dispelling myths and encouraging intervention. *Nurse Practitioner, 14*(5), 47–58.

Kurz, D. (1987). Emergency department responses to battered women: Resistance to medicalization. *Social Problems, 34,* 501–513.

Landenburger, K. (1988). Conflicting realities of women in abusive relationships. In *Communicating nursing research,* (Vol. 21, pp. 15–20).

Landenburger, K. (1989). A process of entrapment in and recovery from an abusive relationship. *Issues in Mental Health Nursing, 10,* 209–227.

Lia-Hoagberg, B., Knoll, K., Swaney, S., Carlson, G., & Mullett, S. (1988). Relationship of street drug use, hospitalization, and psychosocial factors to low birthweight among low income women. *Birth, 15*(1), 8–13.

Lichtenstein, V. R. (1981). The battered woman: Guidelines for effective nursing intervention. *Issues in Mental Health Nursing, 3,* 237–250.

Limandri, B. J. (1986). Research and practice with abused women: Use of the Roy adaptation model as an explanatory framework. *Advances in Nursing Science, 8*(4), 52–61.

Mahon, L. (1981). Common characteristics of abused women. *Issues in Mental Health Nursing, 3,* 137–157.

McFarlane, J., Parker, B., Soeken, K., & Bullock, L., (In press). Abuse during pregnancy: A cross-cultural cohort study of severity and frequency of injuries. *Journal of the American Medical Association.*

O'Brien, J. E. (1971). Violence in divorce prone families. *Journal of Marriage and the Family, 33,* 692–698.

Parker, B., & Schumacher, D. N. (1977). The battered wife syndrome and violence in the nuclear family of origin: A controlled pilot study. *American Journal of Public Health, 67,* 760–761.

Parker, B. (1988). New perspectives on family violence. *Response to the victimization of women and children. 11*(3) 17–19.

Parker, B., & McFarlane, J. (1991). Feminist theory and nursing: An empowerment model for research. *Advances in Nursing Science, 13*(3), 59–67.

Parker, B., Ulrich, Y., Bullock, L., Campbell, D., Campbell, J., King, C., Landenburger, K., McFarlane, J., Ryan, J., Sherdian, D., & Torres, S. (1990). A protocol for safety: Research on the abuse of women. *Nursing Research, 39,* 248–250.

Rose, K., & Saunders, D. G. (1986). Nurses' and physicians' attitudes about women abuse: The effects of gender and professional role. *Health Care for Women International, 7,* 427–438.

Rosenbaum, A. (1988). Methodological issues in marital violence literature. *Journal of Family Violence, 3*(2), 91–104.

Russell, D. (1982). *Rape in marriage.* New York: MacMillan.

Saunders, D. G. (1986). When battered women use violence: Husband abuse or self-defense. *Violence and Victims, 1,* 47–60.

Shipley, S. B., & Sylvester, D. C. (1982). Professionals' attitudes toward violence in close relationships. *Journal of Emergency Nursing, 8*(2), 88–91.

Snell, J., Rosenwald, R., & Robey, A. (1964). The wifebeater's wife. *Archives of General Psychiatry, 11,* 107–112.

Stark, E., Flitcraft, A., Zuckerman, D., Grey, A., Robison, J., & Frazier, W. (1981). *Wife abuse in the medical setting* (Domestic Violence Monograph Series No. 7). Rockville, MD: National Clearinghouse on Domestic Violence.

Straus, M. A., & Gelles, R. J. (1990). *Physical violence in American families.* New Brunswick, NJ: Transaction.

Straus, M. A., Gelles, R. J., & Steinmetz, S. (1980). *Behind closed doors: Violence in American families.* New York: Doubleday.

Stuart, E. P., & Campbell, J. C. (1989). Assessment of patterns of dangerousness with battered women. *Issues in Mental Health Nursing, 10,* 245–260.

Stuart, G., Laraia, M., Ballenger, J., & Lydiard, R. (1990). Early family experiences of women with bulimia and depression. *Archives of Psychiatric Nursing. 4,* 43–52.

Tilden, V. P., & Shepherd, P. (1987). Increasing the rate of identification of battered women in an emergency department: Use of a nursing protocol. *Research in Nursing & Health, 10,* 209–215.

Tolman, R. M., & Bennett, L. W. (1990). A review of quantitative research on men who batter. *Journal of Interpersonal Violence, 5*, 87–118.

Torres, S. (1987). Hispanic-American battered women: Why consider cultural differences? *Responses, 10*(3), 20–21.

Torres, S. (1991). A comparison of wife abuse between two cultures: Perceptions, attitudes, nature and extent. *Issues in Mental Health Nursing. 12*, 113–131.

Trimpey, M. L. (1989). Self-esteem and anxiety: Key issues in an abused women's support group. *Issues in Mental Health Nursing, 10*, 297–308.

Ulrich, Y. (1991). Women's reasons for leaving spouse abuse. *Health Care for Women International. 12*(4), 465–473.

Uphold, C. R., & Strickland, O. L. (1989). Issues related to the unit of analysis in family nursing research. *Western Journal of Nursing Research, 11*, 405–417.

Van Hasselt, V., Morrison, R., Bellack, A., & Hersen, M. (1988). *Handbook of family violence*. New York: Plenum Press.

Walker, L. E. (1979). *The battered woman*. New York: Harper & Row.

Wardell, L., Gillespie, D. L., & Leffler, A. (1983). *Science and violence against wives*. In R. J. Gelles, G. T. Hotaling, M. A. Straus, & D. Finklehor (Eds.), *The dark side of families*, (pp. 69–84). Beverly Hills, CA: Sage.

Weingourt, R. (1990). Wife rape in a sample of psychiatric patients. *Image: Journal of Nursing Scholarship, 22*, 144–147.

Westra, B., & Martin, H. (1981). Children of battered women. *Maternal-Child Nursing Journal, 10*, 41–54.

Yllo, K., & Bograd, M. (1988). *Feminist perspectives on wife abuse*. Newbury Park, CA: Sage.

Chapter 5

Chronic Mental Illness

JEANNE C. FOX
SCHOOL OF NURSING
UNIVERSITY OF VIRGINIA

CONTENTS

Demarcation of chronic mental illness as a research area is difficult for two reasons, one related to the nature of the practice and the other to the problem of understanding the uncertainty of chronic mental illness. Jones and Jones (1987) noted that it is difficult to distinguish the observations and behaviors within psychiatric nursing from those within other mental health professions. More frequently than in other health areas, mental health practitioners across disciplines—medicine, psychiatry, psychology, nursing, and social work—share and interchange roles, tasks, and responsibilities.

The field of psychiatric nursing evolved from psychiatry, nursing, and social sciences. From the middle 1950s well into the 1970s, under the leadership of Peplau and other expert psychiatric nurse educator-practitioners, psychiatric nursing theory and practice reflected interpersonal–intrapsychic paradigms. During this period, psychiatric nurses were primarily concerned with processes of effective interpersonal interventions. For some psychiatric nurses, clinical investigations (research) were focused on the application of psychoanalytic principles and interpretations in psychiatric and general nursing practice. Other nurse practitioner-investigators applied and adapted interpersonal, milieu, and behavioral theories in both individual and group interventions in an effort to improve psychiatric nursing care. Reports of psychiatric nursing research, while infrequent, clearly reflected prevailing psychiatric paradigms.

With the emergence of nursing theories, deinstitutionalization of the 1970s, and recent recognition of the importance of biologic neurostructural factors related to psychiatric illness, the focus of psychiatric nursing research is changing. The care of individuals experiencing mental illness is the core of psychiatric nursing. The perceptual-cognitive, behavioral, emotional, and relational aspects of the life experience of the mentally ill constitute the main concern of the psychiatric nurse. These aspects of mental illness are difficult to demarcate because of the variety of factors affecting these phenomena. Biologic, neurochemical, and cognitive changes can result from physiologic as well as psychologic limitations and disabilities and can influence perceptual, emotional, behavioral, and relationship aspects of the lives of the mentally ill. The domain of psychiatric nursing research is concerned with clients' perception, cognition behavior, emotion, sense of comfort, safety, and health status, in the context of mental illness. However, this review reveals that psychiatric nurse investigators primarily address psychosocial rather than physiologic factors related to chronic mental illness.

Mental health professionals are far from consensus about the meaning of chronic mental illness. Bachrach (1988) suggested that the current ambiguous interpretation of "chronic mental illness" has led investigators either to define chronic mental illness in vague terms or to avoid any definition at all. For purposes of this review, the "chronically mentally ill" are defined, following the Checklist for Chronic Mental Illness Determination (1979), as those persons whose emotional or behavioral functioning is so impaired as to interfere grossly with their capacity to remain in the community without supportive treatment or services of a long-term or indefinite duration. The mental disability is severe and persistent, resulting in long-term limitation of their functional capacities for primary activities of daily living such as interpersonal relationships, homemaking and self-care, employment, or recreation. Diagnoses 295 through 301 in the DSM-III (American Psychiatric Association, 1980), which include such designations as schizophrenic disorders, affective disorders, and personality disorders, are included as qualifying conditions.

LITERATURE REVIEW METHODS

This is a review of psychiatric nursing research on chronic mental illness reported between 1980 and 1989 in the following journals: *Archives in Psychiatric Nursing; Advances in Nursing Science; Image: Journal of Nursing Scholarship; International Journal of Nursing Studies; Issues in Mental Health Nursing; Journal of Advanced Nursing; Journal of Psychosocial Nursing; Nursing Papers; Nursing Research; Perspectives in Psychiatric Nursing; Research in Nursing and Health; Western Journal of Nursing Research; Community Mental Health Journal;* and *Hospital and Community Psychiatry*.

A review of all tables of contents of the journals was conducted, and all research articles related to chronic mental illness that were authored or co-authored by nurses (as determined by published credentials) during the specified time frame were reviewed. Of the 400 psychiatric nursing references reviewed, less than 30 were reports of research on chronic mental illness.

The articles that fell within the demarcated research area were assessed to determine: purpose of study, conceptual framework, study design, population description, sample criteria and size, subject attrition, data-collection procedures, use of standardized instruments, data analysis, and reported findings. The research is reported under the following topics: community adjustment and intervention, recidivism, case management, client self-monitoring and patient education, verbal–nonverbal communication, violence and seclusion, medication compliance, rural service use, and cultural compatibility.

COMMUNITY ADJUSTMENT AND INTERVENTION

Flaskerud (1986a) described 160 chronically mentally ill clients served by four community mental health centers, each of which predominantly cared for a different ethnic/racial community (black, Mexican, Asian, and white). Approximately 52% of the sample were diagnosed as schizophrenic. Systematic record sampling was used to retrieve data from patient records on a standardized form. Flaskerud documented significant relationships between diagnoses of chronic psychoses and gender, marital status, family income, employment, and ethnicity of the clients, as well as frequency of medical problems and treatment, social problems, type of therapy received, discipline of therapist, and pharmacotherapy prescribed. Psychotic clients on medication with medical problems were more likely to see psychiatrists and psychiatric nurses than other therapists.

Although this investigator comprehensively reported client characteristics, there is no information about the community mental health organizations, staffing patterns, case load assignment procedures, or ethnicity of therapists; therefore, conclusions about why psychiatric patients who were chronically mentally ill were more likely to be referred to psychiatrists or psychiatric nurses are speculation. Additional methodologic problems included the absence of a description of how diagnoses were established, absence of subject treatment history, and the likelihood of unexplored interaction of uncontrolled variables.

Ulin (1981) tested the reliability and validity of the Psychological Mental Health Index (PMHI) (Dupuy, 1974) with 108 chronic psychotic adult clients of an urban mental health center. Criteria for inclusion and the process of sample selection were described. Reported reliability and validity of the Mental Health Index were carefully reviewed. Data were collected by social workers and counselors administering the Davis Daily Living Questionnaire and subjects independently completed the Index. In addition, counselors administered the Multi-State Information System Symptom Rating (MSIS) (Lasha et al., 1972), the Overall Symptom Severity Rating (OSS) (Edwards, 1974), and the Counselor's Assessment of Overall Adjustment (COA) (Edwards, 1974). Data were collected at two time periods within a 3-month interval. Concurrent validity was tested with four other measures and the repeated administration generated test–retest reliability. Additional sociodemographic factors and illness-related factors were included to test their effects on scale scores.

The Known Group technique for construct validation was applied by comparing Psychological Mental Health Index scores of the sample with two other sets of scores known to discriminate levels of mental health status, the National Health Survey (Dupuy, 1974) group and the Edwards (1974) client group. Mental Health Index scores for Ulin's (1981) sample of chronically psychotic individuals at admission to the center were significantly lower than the National Health Survey comparison group but higher than the Edwards clients. Limitations of the Psychological Mental Health Index for use with chronically ill subjects were outlined. According to Ulin, this index was capable of discriminating between chronically ill and nonpatient populations. However, chronic psychotics scored higher in subjective well-being than did other mental health intake clients. The Index and the comparison measures demonstrated a consistent relationship to mental health status, but the coefficients were too low to constitute evidence of concurrent validity. A low test–retest coefficient may have reflected instability of the variable in the population or highlighted the inaccuracy of the instrument in measuring change.

This was a generally well-designed investigation. However, criteria for sample selection seriously limited the participation of subjects representative of the population of chronically mentally ill individuals. Therefore, generalizability of findings to this population is not possible.

Stickney, Hall, and Gardner (1980) reported a 4-year prospective investigation designed to assess the effects of four predischarge formats on follow-up compliance and recidivism. Subjects were 400 psychiatric patients discharged consecutively from a state hospital and referred to a specific community mental health center (CMHC); 75.5% were diagnosed as chronic schizophrenics. One hundred patients each were assigned to one of four predischarge conditions: (a) minimum involvement with aftercare consultation (patient at discharge was given phone number of CMHC); (b) an aftercare nurse interviewed patients in the hospital, explained services available at the center, and instructed the patient whom to call; (c) the patient was given a specific appointment as well as the name, address, and number of the aftercare nurse and center, but the aftercare nurse did not interview subjects; and (d) patients were interviewed by the aftercare nurse in the hospital and a specific appointment was set at the CMHC. Aftercare compliance was measured by the patient keeping the initial follow-up appointment. Recidivism was defined as decompensation in mental state that could not be treated with local resources and measured by rehospitalization at the state facility within the year following discharge.

Subjects in the minimum involvement group reflected a 22% rate of compliance and 57% rehospitalization rate. Personal contact before discharge increased compliance by 14%, and specifically scheduling the appointment increased compliance most significantly, from 22% to 68%. The combination of a predischarge interview and appointment scheduling more than tripled compliance from 22% to 75%. Rehospitalization rates between the minimum treatment group and the fourth group were reduced from nearly 57% to 28%, a reduction of one half.

Findings in this investigation supported the importance of structure for effective discharge. However, there is inadequate information about: (a) patient demographics, (b) prior treatment, (c) criteria for formulating diagnoses, (d) community living situations, (e) other factors that may have affected outcomes, and (f) assignment of subjects to discharge treatments. Additionally, the description of data analysis is unclear.

Slavinsky and Krauss (1982) conducted an experimental investigation with a two-group before and after design of two approaches to managing long-term psychiatric outpatients. Forty-seven patients who met clearly specified criteria related to chronic mental illness were assigned randomly to a social support treatment or a medication clinic treatment. The social support approach included medication maintenance plus group intervention. The medication clinic approach did not include psychosocial group support. Subjects were representative of chronically mentally ill populations, and information was presented on subjects' age, marital status, gender, and diagnoses. Investigators reported that despite random assignment, pretreatment assessment of the two groups revealed some significant differences between groups in living and working conditions.

Data on each subject were collected by an investigator using a rating scale in two home visits, at 1 and 2 years in treatment. Information obtained included occupational ratings, socialization ratings, satisfaction with life situation, satisfaction with care, symptom ratings, and motor agitation. Acceptable reliability was reported. Validity was tested by comparison with other established rating tools and psychiatrists' ratings of the Brief Psychiatric Rating Scale (BPRS) (Overall & Gorham, 1962). Patient charts provided documentation of medication increase, rehospitalization, number of days out of the hospital, and treatment dropout.

At the end of the first year of the study, patients in the social support group reported themselves as improved in occupational roles (although those roles had not changed), whereas medication group clients rated themselves lower in occupational roles. Patients in the medication group reported greater satisfaction with care than support group patients. After 2 years, 32 of the original 47 subjects (18 from the support group and 14 from the medication clinic) were interviewed. Thirty-seven percent of the sample had been hospitalized sometime during the 2 years, but there was no statistically significant difference between rehospitalization or total days in the hospital between the two groups. Medication group subjects improved in social adjustment as defined by place of residence and social relating. Medication group clients significantly increased their information-seeking activities (radio, newspaper, television, meetings, contact with neighbors) over pretreatment status, whereas social support group members did not. No difference was reported on life satisfaction of group members, but medication clinic subjects rated their care as contributing a lot to their satisfaction, whereas social group subjects reported care as being somewhat helpful.

The investigators discussed limitations of their findings and design flaws. They noted that treatment integrity as it influences experimental conditions is difficult to assess and control unless the treatment under study is extremely simple. Other research tends to support their finding that medication intervention without social intervention was more acceptable to long-term chronically mentally ill clients than medication indication combined with social group intervention.

RECIDIVISM

Hicks (1989) investigated recidivism with 30 newly readmitted psychiatric patients (20 men, 10 women). Soon after readmission, each subject was interviewed regarding the most recent period between hospitalizations. One hundred twenty-seven interviews were recorded, transcribed, indexed, and catalogued. A content analysis of the qualitative data was conducted. Emerging themes and patterns yielded rich descriptions of subjects' definitions of circumstances, thoughts, and feelings from their most recent community stays. Descriptive statistics were reported for eight major categories: living arrangements, employment, finances, social situation, knowledge and use of community facilities, compliance with discharge plan, other events and reactions, and factors related to community tenure. Gender, age, education, and marital status of the subjects were reported.

Seventeen informants (57%) returned to the hospital in less than 6 months. Thirteen (43%) remained in the community for more than 6 months but less than a year. It was apparent from the findings that subjects led stressful, impoverished lives. Inability to cope with problems related to role transition, living arrangements, and financial concerns were documented. The qualitative design and interpretative method of this investigation were clearly specified. Although such investigations increase our understanding of specific patients' experiences, it is difficult to generalize from them.

Chafetz (1988) reported on her pilot investigation of 77 recidivist clients who utilized walk-in services or emergency rooms and had been hospitalized three times in a year or two times in 6 months. Clinical records provided the major source of this data. Brief interviews with case managers (4) were conducted at the end of the data-collection period to complete and/or verify information from records. Case managers were asked to complete functional rating scales for their clients, using the Uniform Client Data Instrument (UCDI) (Tessler & Mandersheed, 1982) developed by the Federal Community Support Program. The UCDI measures demographic and clinical data, functional status, level of disability, adaptation to community living, and service use. Other characteristics such as homelessness also were assessed.

The investigator documented profiles of subjects, their living situation, and treatment. Findings were that case management services did not have an appreciable impact on the use of emergency services. Although increased length of case management was related to decreasing length of hospital stay, this trend was not statistically significant. Limitations of the study were the small convenience sample and the absence of a comparison group of subjects receiving no case management.

CASE MANAGEMENT

Goering, Waslenki, Farkas, Lancee, and Ballantyre (1988) studied eight case managers in four treatment settings and 88 of the managers' clients. The eight case managers, who were trained in community service coordination skills before the project began, worked out of inpatients units, carried client loads of 15 to 20 patients, and functioned as rehabilitation specialists. In this role, case managers carried out rehabilitation assessments, developed rehabilitation plans, linked patients with community services, monitored patient progress, and acted as a patient advocate. Subjects were selected from all patients admitted to a community rehabilitation service for a 6-month period and screened according to the following criteria: a chronic illness, poor employment history, social isolation, and residential instability. A limited number of patients meeting the criteria were randomly selected to participate in the program. Subjects were matched (for gender, hospital setting, number of previous admissions, diagnosis, and employment status) with comparison subjects who were participants in a citywide study of aftercare. The two groups did not differ significantly in any other demographic or clinical characteristics as far as could be determined. Subjects' diagnoses, history of previous admissions, and marital status were reported.

A survey instrument was administered four times at 6-month intervals. At 24 months, family, patient, or therapists were interviewed by a trained interviewer using the Brief Psychiatric Follow-up Rating Scale (Overall & Gorham, 1962). The study variables of occupational functioning, housing status, and social isolation were defined clearly by the investigators.

Two years after discharge, subjects in the program were significantly higher in occupational functioning than the control group. More subjects in the program were in the high-functioning group and fewer were in the low- and moderate-functioning groups compared with the control subjects. There was no difference in employment status, but more case-managed subjects lived in independent housing. Investigators concluded that rehabilitation case management had a significant impact on client adaptation. Differences in comparison group and case management group use of vocational, housing, social, recreational, and financial services at 6 months post hospitalization were noted. Case-managed subjects used significantly more services, but rehospitalization was not decreased, a finding consistent with other studies of case management—that increased service use does not affect hospitalization rate. An absence of information about medication history and pharmacotherapy during the investigation, for both subjects and comparisons, was a limitation of the study.

CLIENT SELF-MONITORING AND PATIENT EDUCATION

McCandless-Glimcher and associates (1986) interviewed 62 outpatient schizophrenic or schizoaffective subjects in two community mental health centers to determine if schizophrenic subjects recognized symptoms of decompensation and what they did about the symptoms. The Chronic Mental Illness Symptom Interview (Leventhal, Noren, & Strauss, 1982), an adapted instrument, was used to determine whether subjects could tell when they were getting better or worse and what indicators subjects used to make this determination. Subjects also were asked what they did if indicators suggested a worsening of their illness and who assisted them in identifying indicators.

Of the subjects surveyed, 98% claimed that they could tell when they were getting worse, and 89% identified particular symptoms as the chief indicators of a worsening condition. Ninety percent indicated that they could tell when they were getting better, but indicators of improvement were less specific than those associated with getting worse. When symptoms indicated a worsening condition, 58% reported self-treatment (self-medication, engaging in diversionary activity, or ignoring symptoms) and 82% indicated that self-modifying behavior (including self-treatment and assistance seeking) was helpful. No significant relationship was found between self-treatment, seeking assistance, or both, and clients' level of functioning. This investigation addressed a critical aspect of the experience of mental illness. The small convenience sample limits generalizability to other groups.

Youssef (1987) reported an investigation in which 30 patients and their families were involved in an educational program that met twice a week for at least three consecutive sessions. The teaching program was aimed at increasing family knowledge about mental illness, hospitalization, decompensation, and community resources. The investigator measured the effect of family-patient teaching on patient functional level and readmission rate. Subjects were assigned randomly to a family-patient education group or a control group. Subjects were rated before the beginning of the investigation and one year after it with the Global Assessment Scale (GAS), (Endicott, Spitzer, Fliess, & Cohen, 1976, personal communication) and were interviewed about self-knowledge of their psychiatric condition. Youssef reported that the educational program significantly affected scores on the GAS but not readmission of clients. Small sample size and inadequate information about treatment history and community living situations were limitations of the study.

VERBAL AND NONVERBAL COMMUNICATION

Hardin (1980) reported a comparative analysis of verbal and nonverbal communication of schizophrenics and normal subjects. Twelve women were selected purposively and assigned to one of three dyad types: (a) schizophrenic-schizophrenic; (b) schizophrenic-normal; and (c) normal-normal. Subjects' interactions were videotaped for 30 minutes and a previously selected set of nonverbal behaviors were recorded at 1-second intervals. Frequency and duration scores for the sets of nonverbal behaviors with corresponding communication meanings were totaled. The pairs in the three groups differed significantly in engagement with each other and defensiveness. Normal-to-normal dyads were least imitative of each other. The investigator suggested that these findings support the theory of dysjunctive communication in schizophrenia. Dysjunctive communication is the lack of synchrony and involvement, an inability to decipher nonverbal communication of certain affective states, and the use of conflicting and confusing nonverbal cues. The findings provide confirmation of observed deficits in schizophrenic social-perceptual behavior.

PATIENT VIOLENCE AND SECLUSION

Morrison (1989) evaluated a proposed nursing theoretical model in a study of assault and violent episodes in psychiatric settings serving chronically mentally ill clients. Data were collected on 57 nursing staff and 162 hospitalized patients in four hospitals. The investigator found that: (a) inconsistencies in the social and therapeutic rules predicted 18% of the violent behavior and (b) the demographic and medical variables most frequently correlated with violence were history of violence toward others, length of hospitalization, and a diagnosis of substance abuse. The investigator identified a need to link research findings about violence in general with violence in inpatient settings.

Binder and McCoy (1983), over an 8-month period, conducted a study of all patients (24) secluded on a locked ward within one week after their release from that seclusion. Subjects consistently reported that they did not know why they were secluded nor did they know the frequency of staff checks while they were in seclusion. Most reported that nothing was good about the seclusion experience. Only four expressed an appreciation for the therapeutic value of seclusion, and half reported that seclusion had not been necessary. Patients who had been secluded also reported negative attitudes toward the seclusion of others.

Investigators discussed the clinical implications of patients' reports. This study has limited generalizability because of design, sample, and limited use of statistical analysis. However, patient perceptions of their experience could suggest important topics for research related to seclusion.

MEDICATION COMPLIANCE

Youssef (1984) reported an investigation of 126 male and 10 female patients receiving oral medication who were scheduled for discharge from an inpatient facility in 1 month. The purpose of the study was to examine the effect of patient education on medication compliance. Patients were randomly assigned to a patient education group or a control group. The patient education group met twice a week and were provided structured information about drug action, the importance of taking medication, side effects, and reasons for noncompliance. The control group did not meet in education groups and received routine treatment. The length of hospitalization for the two groups differed slightly. Both groups were followed in the community, and compliance was measured by pill count and attendance at follow-up appointments at a mental health clinic. The experimental group had a significantly higher medication compliance at 6 months than did the control group.

The effect of patient education on medication compliance is important. The paucity of information about the treatment history, community experience, and ongoing therapy involvement of the subjects are gaps in the information provided, but random assignment of subjects in this study increases the probability that patient education effect was valid.

Davidhizer (1982a) explored compliance of schizophrenics with medication regimens and described the development of an instrument based on the Fishburn expectancy model to assess the attitude of clients with schizophrenia toward medication. In a second publication this investigator (Davidhizer, 1982b) described factors that have been correlated with compliance for inpatients.

In a 1984 investigation using the above-described instrument, Davidhizer studied patients' beliefs, feelings, and insights about taking medication. The subjects were two groups of 50 consecutive admissions to an acute care psychiatric unit a year apart. The same subject characteristics were described as in the previous investigation.

In 1986 Davidhizer, Austin, and McBride reported an investigation of schizophrenic patients' attitudes toward taking medication. Fifty subjects with schizophrenia were selected from patients consecutively admitted to an acute-care psychiatric unit. All patients were interviewed within the first month of being hospitalized. Each subject responded to questions on three instruments: an open-ended attitude instrument, administered first; a fixed-response attitude instrument, with 26 belief statements, constructed by the investigator from a review of the compliance literature (Davidhizer 1982a) and modified after a pilot study; and an insight instrument. Forty-eight percent of the patients in this study met the criterion for having insight into their disorder. Insight and positive attitude were found to be related. Implications for practice were discussed by the investigators, as were limitations of the study.

Davidhizer's well-developed investigative interest in schizophrenic individuals' compliance is represented in numerous research reports. His work represents a sound qualitative thread in psychiatric-nursing research.

Kucera-Bozarth, Beck, and Lyss (1982) conducted an investigation of 37 adult clients on lithium carbonate who attended public outpatient psychiatric clinics. Demographic data, medication data, and diagnoses were determined from client records. Three self-administered instruments—a medication side effect inventory, the Multidimensional Health Locus of Control Survey (MHLC) (Wallston & Wallston, 1978), and the Health Value Survey—were completed by subjects at their first appointment. Compliance was measured by: (a) appearance at the second of two successive aftercare appointments, (b) deviation scores of two successive serum lithium level assays, and (c) responses to the Self-Reported Lithium Compliance measure (Kucera-Bozarth et al., 1982). Differences between compliant and noncompliant groups were reported. However, this was a sample of convenience and there may well have been numerous uninvestigated factors that influenced noncompliance.

Kurucz and Fallon (1980) investigated dose reduction and discontinuation of antipsychotic medication on a 30-bed inpatient psychiatric unit. Fifteen subjects met the selection criteria, which included diagnosis of chronic schizophrenia, at least 5 years of continuous hospitalization, and present medication not in excess of a daily dose of 300 mg of chlorpromazine or its equivalent. In addition, the subjects could not have required seclusion, intramuscular medication, or increased dosages of medication in the previous 60 days. Age and length of hospitalization were reported.

Medication withdrawal was implemented in two dose-reduction steps within 10 days. Medication was not replaced with placebo, and patients were informed of prescription changes. Medication was reinstated to 50% of its original level if a patient's condition deteriorated, as measured by sporadic maladjustment. No other therapeutic changes were implemented. The Brief Psychiatric Rating Scale (BPRS) (Overall & Gorham, 1962) and the Nurses' Observation Scale (NOSIE) (Honigfeld, Gillis, & Klett, 1966) were used at periodic intervals to assess the patients' condition. The patients whose medication had to be replaced were much younger and had shorter periods of hospitalization. Thirty percent of the patients were still off medication and in good condition at one year.

Clinical implications of these findings were reported by investigators. The absence of a comparison group in this study contributes to a lack of clarity about the meaning of the findings. However, the need for investigation of medication dose reduction and discontinuation remains an important topic for psychiatric nursing research.

Whall, Engle, Edwards, Bobel, and Haberland (1983) reported on the development of a screening program for tardive dyskinesia. A random sample of four aftercare homes was drawn from a sampling frame constructed from a list of 28 homes provided through a metropolitan area community mental health board. The aftercare homes were protected living accommodations for long-term mentally ill individuals discharged to the community; they provided semi-independent living arrangements. Criteria for subject selection were clearly reported as well as subjects' age, gender, length of hospitalization, and medication history. A sample of 60 subjects participated in the study. The purpose of the study was to develop a method of screening in aftercare homes that was valid, reliable, and acceptable to aftercare residents. Four registered nurses who were trained raters conducted client ratings. The Abnormal Involuntary Movement Scale (AIMS) (National Institute of Mental Health, 1976) was utilized to detect tardive dyskinetic movements. Reliability and validity of the AIMS were discussed.

Investigators reported that an acceptable, valid, and reliable screening program was developed. Rater training was highlighted as essential for a successful screening project. This was a comprehensively and rigorously developed feasibility study.

RURAL SERVICE USE

Flaskerud and Koriz (1982) examined health resources that rural community members indicated they would use for specific mental health needs. The study population included all counties classified as rural in six states. Five rural counties were purposively selected from each of the six states for a total of 30 counties. A stratified, statistical probability sample of households in these counties was selected from the most current telephone directories. In addition, in each of the five Illinois counties an independent random sample of households was selected from field listings that were obtained following a multistage selection of places, census tracts, and blocks (or rural segments) with probabilities proportionate to the number of housing units in each county. Data were collected by means of a standardized mailed questionnaire and personal interviews. The return rate of completed questionnaires was 64.5%. Personal interviews were conducted in the five Illinois counties, with an interview response rate of 85.7%. The final combined sample consisted of 367 respondents.

A respondent's choice of help for a specific problem of mental illness was not consistently related to any particular sample characteristic, service, or attitude. Use of general or family practitioners was a preferred choice for some problems but not for all. Flaskerud reported weak associations between choice of a general practitioner for some mental illness problems and quantity and availability of general practitioners. Availability, quantity of service, quality of service, and need for service were not related to any of the other health services. Psychiatrists were identified as a source of care by a majority of respondents for suicidal behavior, hallucinations, and delusions. Implications for community mental health practice were discussed.

The survey data from the Flaskerud and Koriz study (1982) provides a good foundation for planning rural mental health services. However, given the cultural and geographic variations that exist across the United States, it may not be reasonable to generalize these findings to all other rural populations such as those of the rural Southeast.

CULTURAL COMPATIBILITY

Flaskerud (1986b) also reported an investigation of the effects of culture-compatible interventions on the utilization of mental health services by minorities. The records of 300 clients (23.9% Mexican, 22.8% white, 18.1% black, 17.1% Vietnamese, 14.8% Filipino) at four public community health agencies in southern California provided the cases for this study. A systematic sampling frame was established, and 50 records were chosen from each of four agencies, each of which represented one of the ethnic groups. Data were gathered from subjects' clinical records on standardized forms. Specific individual data collected, data-collection procedures, and study variables were thoroughly described by the investigator. Agency and community data related to racial/ethnic factors and formal and informal service utilization also were collected through interviews with staff and the clinical directors, agency records, and census information.

Agencies were given a culture-compatibility score ranging from 1 to 9, with a low score indicating a low level of culture compatibility. Culture compatibility included characteristics such as language and ethnic match, and agency location in an ethnic/racial community. The Asian agency scored highest with a culture-compatibility score of 8.05, the Mexican agency was next with a score of 7.20, the white/mixed agency next with a score of 6.95, and the black agency lowest with a score of 6.00. There were no significant correlations between total culture-compatibility score and dropout status or any single one of the culture-compatibility components and dropout status. A discriminant analysis was done to predict dropout status based on culture-compatibility variables. Standardized discriminant coefficients revealed that three culture-compatibility variables—language match of therapist and client, ethnic/racial match of therapist and client, and agency location in the ethnic/racial community—made the greatest contribution in determining the discriminate score; all other variables were of minor importance. Those three factors were the best predictors of dropout status. Education, previous treatment, and a diagnosis of psychosis were significantly related to remaining in therapy, as was the use of pharmacotherapy in the treatment regimen.

Flaskerud discussed factors that may have contributed to the absence of a definitive relationship between a culturally compatible approach or any of the cultural-compatible components and utilization as measured by dropout status. These factors included difficulties in selecting samples, difficulty of measuring cultural compatibility, and limitations of records as data sources. Flaskerud's comprehensive analysis of culture compatibility provides a good foundation for further studies.

SUMMARY AND RECOMMENDATIONS

Reports of research reviewed for this publication reflected a strong trend of qualitative, ethnomethodologic, and case study investigations. A client-experienced view of phenomena of concern in psychiatric nursing is important. However, the limited reporting of quantitative designs, instrumentation, and data analyses suggests serious gaps in the scientific development of the specialty. Jones and Jones (1987) reported that the scientific rigor of psychiatric nursing research has improved, and it is likely that the quality of psychiatric nursing investigations will continue to improve as more nurses are trained as researchers.

Pfeiffer (1990) identified common recurring weaknesses in psychiatric clinical research publications. These also characterize the psychiatric nursing research on chronic mental illness reviewed by this author. According to Pfeiffer (1990), seven methodologic features are essential and should be reported in descriptions of clinical research: (a) statistical tests used, (b) comparison groups, (c) sample size, (d) subject attrition, (e) blind analyses, (f) adequate dependent measures, and (g) adequate independent measures. Additionally, patient populations should be adequately described in reference to: (a) demographic characteristics, (b) prior treatment, (c) psychiatric diagnoses, (d) criteria for formulating diagnoses, and (e) subdivision of samples.

As other reviewers have reported, the use of statistical analyses is improving in psychiatric nursing research. However, use of control or comparison groups, adequate sample size, and thorough population description did not generally characterize the research reviewed. Given the multiplicity of factors apparently influencing the experiences of individuals with chronic mental illness, it is surprising that multiple regression, path analysis, and modeling methodologies were absent in the research literature reviewed.

Priorities for psychiatric nursing research include investigations of: (a) psychiatric nursing interventions designed to decrease clients' vulnerability to illness experiences or to increase clients' and families' functioning and capacity to cope given the cognitive, information processing, social, and health functioning disabilities associated with schizophrenia and other serious mental illnesses; (b) environmental interventions (including structured living environment treatment systems and community support) designed to compensate for disabilities accompanying schizophrenia and other serious mental illness; (c) alternative models for cost-effective psychiatric and physical health care delivery for individuals and families susceptible to or suffering from mental illness; and (d) psychiatric nursing interventions linking basic research findings with clients' everyday functioning and need for nursing care.

Psychiatric nursing investigators must assume responsibility for advanced knowledge about neurostructural, cognitive, and neurochemical characteristics of individuals experiencing mental illness in addition to knowledge about daily life experience and social-behavioral experiences. Improvement of psychiatric nursing care of mentally ill individuals and survival of psychiatric nursing as a discipline requires increased collaboration of psychiatric nurse researchers with other nursing specialists such as neurologic nurses as well as nonnursing-related basic and behavioral investigators.

REFERENCES

American Psychiatric Association. (1980). *Diagnostic and statistical manual of mental disorders* (3rd ed.). Washington, DC: Author.

Bachrach, L. (1988). Defining chronic mental illness: A concept paper. *Hospital and Community Psychiatry, 39,* 383–388.

Binder, B., & McCoy, S. (1983). A study of patients' attitudes toward placement in seclusion. *Hospital and Community Psychiatry, 34,* 1052–1053.

Carpenter, W. T., Shauss, J. S., & Mulch, S. (1975). Are there pathognomic symptoms in schizophrenia? An empiric investigation of Schneider's first rank symptoms. *Archives of General Psychiatry, 28,* 842–852.

Checklist for chronic mental illness determination. (1979). Phoenix: Arizona Department of Health Services, Division of Behavioral Health Services.

Chafetz, L. (1988). Recidivist clients: A review of pilot data. *Archives in Psychiatric Nursing, 2*(1), 14–20.

Davidhizer, R. (1984). Beliefs and values of the client with chronic mental illness regarding treatment. *Issues in Mental Health Nursing, 6,* 261–275.

Davidhizer, R. (1982a). Compliance by persons with schizophrenia: A research issue. *Issues in Mental Health Nursing, 4,* 233–255.

Davidhizer, R. (1982b). Tool development for profiling the attitude of clients with schizophrenia toward their medication using Fishbein's expectancy value model. *Issues in Mental Health Nursing, 4,* 343–357.

Davidhizer, R., Austin, J., & McBride, A. (1986). Attitudes of patients with schizophrenia toward taking medication. *Research in Nursing and Health, 9,* 139–146.

Dupuy, H. (1974, April). *Utility of the National Center for Health Statistics General Well-Being Schedule in the assessment of self-representations of subjective well-being and distress.* Paper presented at the National Conference on the Evaluation of Drug, Alcohol, and Mental Health Programs, Washington, DC.

Edwards, D. W. (1974). *Davis Outcome Assessment System (V2).* Unpublished manuscript University of California at Davis, Department of Psychiatry, Davis.

Flaskerud, J. (1986a). Profile of chronically mentally ill psychotic patients in four community mental health centers. *Issues in Mental Health Nursing, 8*(2), 155–168.

Flaskerud, J. (1986b). The effects of culture-compatible intervention on the utilization of mental health services by minority clients. *Community Mental Health Journal, 22,* 127–141.

Flaskerud, J., & Koriz, F. (1982). Resources rural consumers indicate they would use for mental health problems. *Community Mental Health Journal, 18,* 107–119.

Goering, P., Waslenki, D., Farkas, M., Lancee, W., & Ballantyre, R. (1988). What difference does case management make? *Hospital and Community Psychiatry, 39,* 272–276.

Hardin, S. (1980). Comparative analyses of nonverbal interpersonal communication of schizophrenics and normals. *Research in Nursing and Health, 3,* 57–68.

Hicks, M. (1989). A community sojourn from the perspective of one who relapsed. *Issues in Mental Health Nursing, 10,* 137–147.

Honigfeld, G., Gillis, R. D., & Klett, J. (1966). NOSIE-30: A treatment & sensitive hard behavioral scale. *Psychological Reports, 19,* 180–182.

Jones, S., & Jones, P. K. (1987). Research in psychiatric and mental health nursing: The emergence of scientific rigor. *Archives of Psychiatric Nursing, 1*(3), 155–162.

Kucera-Bozarth, K., Beck, N., & Lyss, L. (1982). Compliance with lithium regimens. *Journal of Psychosocial Nursing and Mental Health Services, 20*(7), 11–15.

Kurucz, J., & Fallon, J. (1980). Dose reduction and discontinuation of antipsychotic medication. *Hospital and Community Psychiatry, 31,* 117–119.

Laska, E. et al. (1972). The multistate information system. *Evaluation, 1,* 66–71.

Leventhal, H., Noren, Z. D., & Strauss, A. (1982). Self-regulation and the mechanism for symptom appraisal in symptoms, illness behavior, and help seeking (D. Mechanic, Ed.). New York: Prodist.

McCandless-Glimcher, L., McKnight, S., Hamera, E., Smith, B., Peterson, K., & Plumber, A. (1986). Use of symptoms by schizophrenics to monitor and regulate their illness. *Hospital and Community Psychiatry, 37,* 929–933.

Morrison, E. (1989). Theoretical modeling to predict violence in hospitalized psychiatric patients. *Research in Nursing and Health, 12,* 31–40.

National Institute of Mental Health. (1976). Abnormal Involuntary Movement Scale. In W. Guy (Ed.), *ECDEU Assessment Manual.* Rockville, MD: U.S. Department of Health, Education, and Welfare.

Overall, J., & Gorham, D. (1962). The Brief Psychiatric Rating Scale. *Psychiatric Reports, 10,* 799–812.

Pfeiffer, S. (1990). An analysis of methodology in follow-up studies of adult inpatient psychiatric treatment. *Hospital and Community Psychiatry, 41,* 1315–1321.

Slavinsky, A., & Krauss, J. B. (1982). Two approaches to the management of long term psychiatric outpatients in the community. *Nursing Research, 31,* 284–289.

Stickney, L., Hall, R., & Gardner, R. (1980). The effect of referral procedures on aftercare compliance. *Hospital and Community Psychiatry, 31,* 567–569.

Tessler, R., & Mandersheed, R. (1982). Factors affecting adjustment to community living: Hospital and community. *Psychiatry, 33,* 203–207.

Ulin, P. (1981). Measuring adjustment in chronically ill Community mental health care. *Nursing Research, 30,* 229–235.

Wallston, K. A., & Wallston, B. S. (1978). Development of the Multidimensional Health Locus of Control (MHLC) Scales. *Health Education Monographs, 6,* 160–170.

Whall, A., Engle, V., Edwards, A., Bobel, L., & Haberland, C. (1983). Development of a screening program for tardive dyskinesia: Feasibility issues. *Nursing Research, 32,* 151–156.

Youssef, F. (1984). Adherence to therapy in psychiatric patients: An empirical investigation. *International Journal of Nursing Studies, 21,* 51–59.

Youssef, F. (1987). Discharge planning for psychiatric patients: The effect of a family patient teaching program. *Journal of Advanced Nursing, 12,* 611–616.

Chapter 6

Alcohol and Drug Abuse in Nurses

Eleanor J. Sullivan
School of Nursing
University of Kansas Medical Center

Sandra M. Handley
School of Nursing
University of Kansas Medical Center

CONTENTS

In this chapter, the research on alcohol and other drug abuse in nurses is reviewed. Using the (DSM-III-R) terminology, the appropriate diagnostic terms for addictive disorders are *psychoactive substance abuse* and *psychoactive substance dependence*. Alcohol abuse, alcohol dependence, and abuse and dependence of specific drugs and dependence are included in these diagnoses (American Psychiatric Association, 1987). *Dependence* is diagnostically defined as impaired control of substance use and continued use despite adverse consequences. *Abuse* is defined as maladaptive patterns of substance use. In this chapter, the terms alcohol and drug abuse and dependence are used even though terminology was not always well defined in the reports.

Research on alcohol and drug abuse in nurses published between 1980 and 1990 is reviewed. Initial data were gathered by a computer search of the

Cumulative Index of Nursing and Allied Health Literature (CINAHL) from 1983 to 1991. The topics searched were substance use, substance dependence, alcohol, and alcoholism. A manual search of CINAHL was conducted for the years 1980 to 1983. Also, the two leading journals in the field, the *Journal of Studies on Alcohol* and the *International Journal of Addictions,* were searched manually for relevant articles by nurse authors. References from current texts in the field were reviewed. The ancestry approach was used to obtain relevant citations from each study reviewed.

The review was limited to published research in which a nurse was first or second author and sufficient methodological detail was reported. Studies of nurses by nonnurse authors were included selectively when those studies represented important contributions to the body of knowledge. Nursing studies from other English-speaking countries, primarily Great Britain and Canada, also were reviewed.

The research was divided into three thematic categories: (a) the prevalence of alcohol and drug abuse in nurses and student nurses; (b) characteristics of nurses who abuse alcohol and drugs; and (c) nurses' attitudes toward colleagues with alcohol or drug dependence problems.

PREVALENCE

In the following studies, researchers attempted to quantify the abuse of alcohol and drugs in nurses and student nurses.

Nurses

Researchers questioned 249 randomly selected registered nurses and licensed practical nurses employed in hospitals in a New Mexico county about the frequency of alcohol and drug use (Smith, Mangelsdorf, Loudersbough, & Piland, 1989). In this sample, alcohol use was more common than other drugs: 6% of the sample used alcohol daily and 22% used it once or twice a week. Tranquilizers, marijuana, and commercial diet pills were used daily by 1% of the sample. The results of this study were difficult to compare with other findings as actual alcohol or drug abuse or dependence cannot be determined by frequency of use data alone without quantity, use patterns, and consequences of use.

Gerace (1988) studied the alcohol use of 160 nurse educators at two Midwestern universities. She used both quantity and frequency data to calculate an annual quantity–frequency index. These data were compared with data on the general population of American women. Nurse educators had fewer abstainers (10% versus 40%), fewer heavy drinkers (1% versus 4%), and more light drinkers (62% versus 38%). Gerace's comparisons suggested that nurses drink more often but not as heavily as other women. Strengths of the study included the use of the annual drinking index, which considers several drinking behaviors; the comparison of nurses with a national sample; and a high return rate (82%). Only alcohol use was examined; other drug-use data were not collected.

Hickman, Finke, and Miller (1990) studied the relationship between alcohol and/or drug use and work behaviors. They surveyed 92 female nurses in one hospital about their alcohol and drug use in the previous month. Use was compared with their errors, accidents, and tardiness or absences at work. They found that 12% drank 3 to 4 days per week and 5% drank 5 or more days per week. When subjects who drank less than twice a week were compared with those who drank three to seven times per week, there were no significant differences in their reported errors, accidents, or absences. Conclusions must be regarded as preliminary, however, because a limited population was sampled and sensitive information (e.g., alcohol and drug use, errors, and work attendance) was collected from self-reports. Use of self-report data limit the reliability of the responses.

Student Nurses

Alcohol and drug use by student nurses have been more extensively studied, probably because of the availability of subjects. McAuliffe et al., (1984) surveyed students in seven professions (medicine, business, law, social work, communications, counseling, and nursing) on their drug use. The student nurse sample consisted of 358 students from five Boston-area nursing schools. In the survey researchers asked only whether specific drugs had *ever been used*. The percentage of student nurses who had ever used specific drugs were as follows: marijuana, 62%; amphetamines, 14%; tranquilizers, 13%; hallucinogens, 9%; sedatives, 5%; and cocaine, 15%. Generally, student drug use was low and nursing student use was lower than any of the other professional student groups. McAuliffe's work was built on his epidemiologic studies of drug use in the professions (McAuliffe et al., 1986, 1991) in which he used acceptably large samples. The most common drug of abuse, alcohol, however, was not included in this work.

Haack and Harford (1984) studied drinking patterns in 179 senior nursing students in one nursing program. Nursing students were more likely to be weekly drinkers than were other college women, and the proportion of student nurses who were heavy drinkers was somewhat higher than for other college students. Of the student nurses, 13% reported that their drinking interfered with their studies or their work. In later work, Haack, Harford, and Parker (1988) also found that a family history of drinking was associated with greater student consumption. Haack and colleagues (1984, 1988) did not include drug use in their surveys. Conclusions are limited by the use of students from one school of nursing and students' self-report data.

Engs has conducted a series of studies of alcohol and drug use in students, including nursing students, both in the United States and abroad. Engs (1982) studied drinking patterns in 1,691 Australian nursing and other human service students (law, medicine, pharmacy, police, seminary, and social work). Overall, 68% (N = 1,691) of the students were considered light drinkers and 3% were heavy drinkers with potential problems. Of the six professional groups, the student nurses (n = 213) ranked fifth in consumption, with only seminary students lower.

Drug use in this sample also was reported (Engs, 1980). No nursing student reported current use of hallucinogens, cocaine, or opiates. However, nursing students were the third highest group in reported current use of sedatives and tranquilizers. Overall, professional students' drug use was slightly less than that of Australian college students in general.

Engs and Rendell (1987) compared first-year (n = 102) nursing students with last-year (n = 107) nursing students to determine changes in alcohol and drug use over the course of the nursing program. There were no differences in frequency or quantity of alcohol consumption between the two groups. Two percent were classified as heavy, or at-risk, drinkers. Another 2% were considered possible problem drinkers. There were no significant differences in the use of analgesics, marijuana, or other drugs between the groups with the exception of amphetamines, which were used more often by first-year students. In the study investigators used a cross-sectional design and did not specifically measure changes in individual students' use. However, this study is unique in its attempt to measure change in alcohol and drug use.

A subsequent study by Engs and Hanson (1989) compared American nursing students' drinking patterns and alcohol knowledge in 1982–1983 (n = 291) and 1984–1985 (n = 170). Although the surveys were used to sample the same population, responses were anonymous and thus unmatched. Over the 2-year period, there were few changes in alcohol knowledge or in drinking patterns or problems. About one-quarter of the students were classified as moderately heavy to heavy drinkers, indicating that alcohol abuse may be more extensive than reported in earlier studies.

Like McAuliffe and colleagues, Engs has established a research program studying addictive problems in student professionals. Engs used volunteer subjects who self-reported information; responses were anonymous and large, diverse sample sizes were appropriate to epidemiologic studies. Additionally, Engs examined prevalence over time and included both alcohol and other drugs.

There is no indication that the prevalence of alcohol or drug abuse in nurses is any higher than in the population as a whole (Gerace, 1988;

Hickman et al., 1990; Smith et al., 1989). Studies are limited, however, by comparatively small sample sizes and circumscribed geographic locations. In the larger, epidemiologic studies of student nurses, the prevalence of alcohol or drug problems is reported as slightly less compared to both professional students (McAuliffe et al., 1984) and other college students (Engs, 1980, 1982).

More recent reports by Haack et al. (1988) and Engs and Hanson (1989), however, suggested that alcohol abuse in nursing students may be increasing. Because students are in an optimal position for learning about the risks involved in alcohol and drug use, it is important to examine this problem in depth. A longitudinal study of students postgraduation and into practice years would yield important data about changes in use over time.

A common methodologic problem in the studies was the variety of measures employed to determine alcohol or drug use. Also, examining alcohol use (Gerace, 1988; Haack & Harford, 1984; Haack, et al., 1988) separate from drug use (McAuliffe et al., 1984) made comparisons difficult and limited opportunities to determine the degree of polydrug use and abuse.

CHARACTERISTICS OF ALCOHOL- AND DRUG-DEPENDENT NURSES

Using retrospective methods, descriptive data have been collected on alcohol- and drug-dependent nurses, frequently termed impaired nurses. These studies have been focused on identifying personal and professional characteristics of nurses whose practice is impaired due to alcohol or drug dependence. Results have been obtained primarily through surveys of nurses who are self-identified as both alcohol or drug dependent and as recovering from dependence.

Descriptive Studies

Bissell and Jones (1981) interviewed 100 recovering alcoholic nurses. Sixty-two percent were dependent on alcohol only, 23% used alcohol as well as other drugs, and 15% reported alcohol and narcotic use. Subjects reported high academic achievement and numerous consequences to their drinking. Few had been sanctioned either by employers or licensing boards. At follow-up interviews 5 to 7 years later, 79% had remained abstinent (Bissell & Haberman, 1984), indicating a high recovery rate. The researchers used a convenience sample of volunteer subjects who self-reported both their addiction and their recovery. This limited the reliability of the results. However, the study was the first description of impaired nurses. It has been frequently cited in subsequent studies and is considered to be influential in the movement to assist impaired nurses.

Reed (1988) interviewed 26 recovering nurses in a Georgia nurse support group. Important findings were: 43% identified their specialty as critical care; 35% had a parent who abused alcohol or drugs; 15% were dependent on alcohol; 46% were dependent on other drugs; and, 39% were dependent on both alcohol and drugs. The conclusions were limited by the small, nonrandom local group. Of interest, however, is the high percentage of critical care nurses and the percentage of combined alcohol and drug use, which is consistent with other studies.

Richeson (1989) reviewed the records for the years 1956 to 1984 of all 122 nurses sanctioned by the Florida licensing board for alcohol or drug abuse. Associate degree graduates appeared to be overrepresented in the sample compared to their percentage in the state (44% versus 37% in 1985). Using records over a 28-year period, however, created historical confounds; for example, the years of the study span the development of associate degree programs. Additionally, the researcher was dependent on the accuracy of previous records collected during times when little was known about alcohol or drug abuse. Because state licensing boards more often sanction for drug use or abuse than for alcohol abuse (Sullivan, Bissell, & Leffler, 1990), it is likely that these data from licensing boards underrepresent alcohol problems in nurses.

Sullivan (1987a) surveyed 139 recovering alcohol- or drug-dependent nurses (self-identified) and found the following characteristics: family histories of alcoholism and depression; personal histories of sexual abuse and dysfunction; and extensive medical histories of medical problems. A larger percentage of subjects were male (12%) than the percentage of males in nursing (3%). In spite of serious problems resulting from their alcohol (43%), drug (23%), or combined alcohol and drug (32%) use, subjects reported professional and academic success. One-third of the sample had used alcohol or drugs since initial recovery but all had returned to abstinence at the time of data collection. Conclusions must be made guardedly because the sample was acquired indirectly through assistance organizations for nurses. Both the response rate and characteristics of nonrespondents were unknown, rendering the representativeness of the sample questionable. Additionally, subjects self-reported both addiction and recovery and no attempt was made to verify either condition. This study was the first to include sexual abuse and problems as a variable in this population (Sullivan, 1988). Given the high percentage of sexual problems reported, additional investigation of the relationship of sexual problems and alcohol and drug abuse are indicated.

Sullivan (1987b) then surveyed 1,000 nurses randomly selected from six state board of nursing rosters; 522 nurses from 18 states responded. After screening for the possibility of alcohol or drug problems, 384 subjects were compared with the dependent nurses in the previous survey. Dependent nurses had a significantly greater incidence of family histories of alcoholism and depression; sexual problems; homosexuality; alcoholic spouses; physical health problems; history of depression; marital breakup; and being male. Limitations of the study include the low response rate (30%) of nondependent subjects, self-selection of dependent nurses, and lack of verification of subjects' addiction or recovery status.

To investigate the effects of drug use on job performance and related disciplinary actions, Sullivan et al. (1990) surveyed a convenience sample of 300 drug-dependent nurses. Using a drug use history, the researchers found that one-fourth of these subjects used drugs prior to nursing school, the majority also were alcohol dependent (77%), and that polydrug use was common. Younger nurses and men more often used narcotics, while older nurses and women more often reported alcohol abuse. Seventy nine percent reported that their drug use affected their job. However, only 23% were sanctioned by the state licensing board. Although methodologic weaknesses (sampling and instrumentation) limit conclusions, such exploratory findings are useful to identify areas of inquiry for future investigation.

Norris, Pierson, and Waugaman (1988) interviewed 21 recovering, certified registered nurse anesthetists (CRNAs) to identify characteristics associated with alcohol and drug abuse in this specialized nurse population. Seventy-six percent reported working under the influence of drugs, particularly when they were on call; only 28% were involved with licensing boards. Most (75%) thought their co-workers knew of their problems and did nothing. A standardized data set would allow comparisons of this special population with the general nurse population.

Qualitative Studies

In four studies researchers used qualitative approaches to examine the impaired nurse. Church (1985) conducted a historical study of articles on alcohol or drug abuse in nurses in the nursing literature from 1900 to 1985. She found only three articles from 1900 to 1955. After 1955, the topic appeared occasionally until the 1970s. Church concluded that alcohol and drug abuse in nurses was historically denied or ignored within the profession until the late 1970s, when members of the American Nurses Association (ANA) began efforts to legitimize assistance for impaired nurses (ANA, 1984).

Hutchinson (1986, 1987) used grounded theory to describe the process of addiction and recovery in impaired nurses. In the first study, she interviewed

20 recovering nurses from a state assistance program (Hutchinson, 1986). The process of addiction was conceptualized as a "trajectory toward self-annihilation" that included the following stages: the early experience with substances; the commitment or decision to "use"; and the eventual compulsion to use which began to control the subject's life. With the same sample, the investigator also described recovery, which was conceptualized as self-integration with stages of surrendering, accepting, and committing (Hutchinson, 1987). While this conceptualization was new to the study of impairment in nurses, the results are similar to other information about alcohol or drug abuse in nurses and the general population. However, this research provided methodologic triangulation in that similar results were achieved through different research methods, therefore verifying the findings. The identification of specific stages is also helpful to those who intervene with impaired nurses.

Stammer (1988) used an ethnographic approach to identify the cultural path toward alcoholism in 34 recovering nurses from one southern state. Stress and tension related to underlying feelings of worthlessness emerged as themes related to the development of alcohol abuse. Disruption in the family of origin and family histories of alcohol or drug abuse were common (80%). Half of the subjects drank heavily during childhood and/or adolescence. Subject descriptions of reentry to nursing practice suggested problems with reentry, and 62% changed work settings after treatment (Stammer, 1989).

It is not clear to what extent this study was truly ethnographic. Data were collected by interview rather than by participant observation techniques characteristic of ethnography. The analysis of data produced both qualitative and quantitative data. The cultural path is broadly described, primarily in family terms, and although indicators of substance use are developed, the origins of these data are unclear.

The findings of Hutchinson (1986, 1987) and Stammer (1988, 1989) were consistent with the data reported in descriptive studies as well as the literature on alcohol and drug abuse. They have added important process dimensions to the literature on impaired and recovering nurses.

Persistent methodologic problems in the studies of impaired nurses included small sample sizes (Norris et al., 1988; Reed, 1988), potential geographic bias (Hutchinson, 1986, 1987; Stammer, 1988, 1989), the use of nurses *recovering* from dependence problems to explain addiction (Bissell & Haberman, 1984; Bissell & Jones, 1981; Hutchison, 1986, 1987; Norris et al., 1988; Reed, 1988; Richeson, 1989; Stammer, 1988, 1989; Sullivan 1987a, 1988; Sullivan et al., 1990), and the representativeness of convenience samples of recovering nurses (Sullivan, 1987a; Sullivan et al., 1990). These methodologic problems highlight the difficulty of locating and accessing a sample of dependent nurses.

NURSES' ATTITUDES TOWARD IMPAIRED COLLEAGUES

Another area of inquiry has been nurses' attitudes toward their colleagues who abuse alcohol and drugs. This has become important as nursing organizations develop peer assistance problems for impaired nurses and as recovering nurses return to the workplace. In three studies researchers have examined these attitudes.

Hendrix, Sabritt, McDaniel, and Field (1987) surveyed 1,047 randomly selected nurses in a southeastern state to determine whether perceptions of impaired nurses differed by respondent's position (administration or staff) or by the type of impairment (alcohol, drug, or emotional distress). Differences in attitudes existed according to respondents' job position. Supervisors favored disciplinary action more often than staff nurses, whereas staff nurses more often believed in the effectiveness of treatment. Differences also were found by type of impairment. Discipline was recommended more often by respondents when impairment was due to alcohol or drug abuse rather than to emotional distress. Strengths of the study included adequate instrument development and testing; use of a large, randomly selected sample; an acceptable response rate (65%); and appropriate multivariate analyses.

Cannon and Brown (1988) surveyed 396 Oregon nurses on their attitudes toward alcoholic and drug-abusing clients and included attitudes toward impaired colleagues. The investigators found that nurses who were more positive toward alcohol and drug use in clients also were more positive toward impaired nurses. In addition, subjects were more positive toward alcohol- (rather than drug-) abusing nurses. The longer the respondent had been employed in nursing practice, the more negative the attitude toward both clients and colleagues. This finding also was suggested by supervisors' negative attitudes in the Hendrix et al. (1987) study. By using systematic sampling and the Substance Abuse Attitude Survey (Chappel, Veach, & Krug, 1985), a standardized instrument for assessing attitudes, these results suggest that the work experience influences nurses' attitudes toward their colleagues.

Lachicotte and Alexander (1990) investigated nurse administrators' attitudes toward nurse impairment and their method of responding to the problem. A small sample (*N* = 36) of South Carolina nurse executives were surveyed using two instruments: the Attitudes Towards Nurse Impairment Inventory (adapted from Tolor & Tamerin, 1975) and the Methods for Dealing with Nurse Impairment Questionnaire (developed by the authors). Subjects more often believed that alcohol or drug abuse was caused by psychologic, physical, or genetic factors rather than moral weakness. Administrators with positive beliefs about etiology more often favored an assistive, rather than punitive, approach. Marginal reliabilities (.35 to .76) of the

Attitudes Toward Nurse Impairment Inventory subscales weaken the conclusions. Also, the researchers did not report the method used to acquire the sample.

These three studies suggested that more experienced nurses and supervisors held more negative and punitive attitudes toward their impaired colleagues. It would be of interest to know how variables such as education, managerial experience, and others affect attitudes. A yet unstudied factor is how experience, either personal or professional, with impaired nurses affects attitudes. These findings have implications for recovering nurses returning to nursing practice.

SUMMARY AND FUTURE DIRECTIONS

The study of prevalence of alcohol and drug problems in nurses and student nurses suggested that nurses do not suffer from these conditions more often than others in society. There is some indication, however, that the younger population of nurses may be more at risk for these disorders.

Although determining characteristics of addicted, recovering nurses is useful in exploring a new research topic, the descriptive studies reported to date are limited. Specifically, this field of study lacks systematic knowledge building and a useful theoretical base. This lack of theory, however, plagues the entire field of alcohol and drug studies. With a few exceptions, there is a lack of programs of research. Studies have not been replicated, nor are they used as the basis for new research. Long-term recovery in nurses has not been studied. There is little exploration of recovery or recovery rates or the variables that facilitate recovery. Such studies would require longitudinal research, which may require more commitment to the topic and more stable funding. Recovery, either spontaneous without treatment or through self-help groups, should be examined. Studying impaired nurses not in recovery is even more difficult and has not been attempted. Reentry to nursing practice is another difficult topic yet to be explored. Also, there is a need for well-designed intervention studies. Nurse-run peer assistance programs may provide access to subjects for such studies. Research also is needed on the impact of early detection and intervention with both students and nurses.

In the limited work to date, nurses' attitudes toward other nurses with addiction problems have been found to be negative. Again, these studies are primarily descriptive. Researchers have not explored the relationship of attitudes to experience. Only Hendrix et al. (1987) collected data on how attitudes related to behavior and those data were collected retrospectively. Intervention studies to impact attitudes have not yet been conducted.

Subject vulnerability helps to explain why so few controlled studies of this problem have been conducted. Nurses are put in jeopardy when their addictions are known to employers and/or state licensing boards. Exceptional precautions must be taken when these nurses participate in research. Investigators are challenged to design well-controlled studies while at the same time protecting these vulnerable subjects.

The stigma attached to alcohol or drug abuse in nurses and the still common denial of the problem within the nursing profession make pursuit of this research difficult. Nurses attempting research in this area have found funding difficult to obtain and publication of results problematic due to attitudes toward the topic.

Increasing societal and professional awareness of alcohol and drug abuse increases the need for research on alcohol and drug abuse in nurses. Mandatory reporting laws have promoted the development of monitored assistance programs for impaired nurses. Such programs increase the availability of information on dependent nurses and provide a potential sampling frame for research. Research on nurses, as a specialized population of women, is needed because it adds to the knowledge base on alcohol and drug abuse in women.

The impact of nursing impairment on clients and public safety, as well as concern for nursing colleagues, mandates that the study of this vulnerable population continue. The need is for nurse researchers committed to the topic and for more rigorous research designs.

REFERENCES

American Nurses' Association. (1984). *Addictions and psychological dysfunction in nursing: The profession's response to the problem*. Kansas City, MO: Author.

American Psychiatric Association. (1987). *Diagnostic and statistical manual of mental disorders* (3rd ed., rev.). Washington, DC: Author.

Bissell, L., & Haberman, P. (1984). *Alcoholism in the professions*. New York: Oxford.

Bissell, L., & Jones, R. W. (1981). The alcoholic nurse. *Nursing Outlook, 29,* 96–101.

Cannon, B. L., & Brown, J. S. (1988). Nurses' attitudes toward impaired colleagues. *Image, 20,* 96–101.

Chappel, J. N., Veach, T. L., & Krug, R. S. (1985). The substance abuse attitude survey: An instrument for measuring attitudes. *Journal of Studies on Alcohol, 46,* 48–52.

Church, O. M. (1985). Sairey Gamp revisited: A historical inquiry into alcoholism and drug dependency. *Nursing Administration Quarterly, 9*(2), 15–19.

Engs, R. C. (1980). The drug-use patterns of helping-profession students in Brisbane, Australia. *Drug and Alcohol Dependence, 6,* 231–246.

Engs, R. C. (1982). Drinking patterns and attitudes toward alcoholism of Australian human-service students. *Journal of Studies on Alcohol, 5,* 517–529.

Engs, R. C., & Hanson, D. J. (1989). Alcohol knowledge and drinking patterns of nursing students over time. *College Student Journal, 23*(1), 82–88.

Engs, R. C., & Rendell, K. H. (1987). Alcohol, tobacco, caffeine and other drug use among nursing students in the Tayside Region of Scotland: A comparison between first- and final-year students. *Health Education Research, 2,* 329–336.

Gerace, L. (1988). Patterns of alcohol use among nurse educators. *Issues in Mental Health Nursing, 9,* 189–200.

Haack, M. R. (1988). Stress and impairment among nursing students. *Research in Nursing and Health, 11,* 125–134.

Haack, M. R., & Harford, T. C. (1984). Drinking patterns among student nurses. *International Journal of the Addictions, 19,* 577–583.

Haack, M. R., Harford, T. C., & Parker, D. A. (1988). Alcohol use and depression symptoms among female nursing students. *Alcoholism: Clinical and Experimental Research, 12,* 365–367.

Hendrix, M. J., Sabritt, D., McDaniel, A., & Field, B. (1987). Perceptions and attitudes toward nursing impairment. *Research in Nursing and Health, 10,* 323–333.

Hickman, L., Finke, L., & Miller, E. (1990). Nurses with chemical dependency: Usage and job performance effects. *Addictions Nursing Network, 2*(1), 14–16.

Hutchinson, S. (1986). Chemically dependent nurses: The trajectory toward self-annihilation. *Nursing Research, 35,* 196–201.

Hutchinson, S. (1987). Toward self-integration: The recovery process of chemically dependent nurses. *Nursing Research, 36,* 339–343.

Lachicotte, J. D., & Alexander, J. W. (1990). Management attitudes and nurse impairment. *Nursing Management, 21*(9), 102–110.

McAuliffe, W. E., Rohman, M., Breer, P., Wyshak, G., Santangelo, S., & Magnuson, E. (1991). Alcohol use and abuse in random samples of physicians and medical students. *American Journal of Public Health, 81,* 177–182.

McAuliffe, W. E., Rohman, M., Santangelo, S., Feldman, B., Magnuson, E., Sobol, A., & Weissman, J. (1986). Psychoactive drug use among practicing physicians and medical students. *New England Journal of Medicine, 315,* 805–810.

McAuliffe, W. E., Wechsler, H., Rohman, M., Soboroff, S. H., Fishman, P., Toth, D., & Friedman, R. (1984). Psychoactive drug use by young and future physicians. *Journal of Health and Social Behavior, 25,* 34–54.

Norris, J., Pierson, F., & Waugaman, W. (1988). Critical factors associated with substance abuse and chemical dependency in nurse anesthesia. *Journal of Alcohol and Drug Education, 33*(2), 6–13.

Reed, M. T. (1988). Descriptive study of chemically dependent nurses, In J. Brooking (Ed.), *Psychiatric Nursing Research* (pp. 157–173). New York: Wiley.

Richeson, M. B. (1989). Substance abusing nurses appearing before the Board of Nursing. *Mississippi RN,* November–December, 14–15.

Smith, H. L., Mangelsdorf, K. L., Louderbough, A. W., & Piland, N. F. (1989). Substance abuse among nurses: Types of drugs. *Dimensions of Critical Care Nursing, 8*(3), 159–169.

Stammer, M. E. (1988). Understanding alcoholism and drug dependency in nurses. *Quality Review Bulletin, 14*(3), 75–80.

Stammer, M. E. (1989). Cultural path effects on chemical dependency and recovery in professional nurses. *Addictions Nursing Network, 1*(4), 17–19.

Sullivan, E. J. (1987a). A descriptive study of nurses recovering from chemical dependency. *Archives of Psychiatric Nursing, 1,* 194–200.

Sullivan, E. J. (1987b). Comparison of chemically dependent and nondependent nurses on familial, personal and professional characteristics. *Journal of Studies on Alcohol, 48,* 563–568.

Sullivan, E. J. (1988). Association between chemical dependency and sexual problems in nurses. *Journal of Interpersonal Violence, 3,* 326–329.

Sullivan, E. J., Bissell, L., & Leffler, D. (1990). Drug use and disciplinary actions among 300 nurses. *International Journal of the Addictions, 25,* 375–391.

Tolor, A., & Tamerin, J. S. (1975). The Attitudes Toward Alcoholism Instrument: A measure of attitudes towards alcoholics and the nature and causes of alcoholism. *British Journal of Addiction, 70,* 223–231.

Chapter 7

Childhood and Adolescent Bereavement

Nancy D. Opie
College of Nursing and Health
University of Cincinnati

CONTENTS

This review of nursing research on childhood and adolescent bereavement covers a relatively short time span (1983 to 1990), reflecting publication of the first nursing research report on childhood bereavement in 1983 (Long, 1983). Bereavement is defined as the state of having lost the relationship of a significant other (parent, sibling, grandparent, etc.) by death. The review is limited to those studies in which researchers investigated bereavement phenomena in children (1 year to 12 years) and adolescents (13 years to 18 years). Studies in which the influence of bereavement on children's and adolescents' health and well-being (behavior, peer and family relationships, physical, emotional, and academic well-being) or which investigated factors effecting the process of grief and mourning were selected for this review. A necessary criterion was that children and adolescents were either the subjects, were included as subjects (e.g., family studies), or were the objects of the data collected (parent provided data about the child). It does not include studies of adult subjects who had sustained a significant loss by death during childhood, nor does it include studies of children's concept of death. This review does not include studies related to loss of self through death, or loss of one's own body parts (e.g., an arm or leg), nor does it include studies related to loss due to divorce, desertion, or incarceration of a significant other.

Several methods were used to retrieve research reports. First, computer searches were conducted of all volumes of the nursing, medical, psychiatric, psychologic, sociologic, thanatologic, and educational literature from 1980 to March 1990. Abstracts of articles were acquired with computer searches. Each citation that gave indication of a nursing author(s) was retrieved. Abstracts and research citations that did not identify the discipline of the author(s) were retrieved and read in a further attempt to identify manuscripts authored by nurses. The reference lists of all articles were scanned for potential articles, books, or chapters written by nurses. A computer search of dissertation abstracts was conducted from 1980 to March of 1990. Previous reviews of bereavement written by nurses (Benoliel, 1983; Betz, 1987; Demi & Miles, 1986; Valente, Saunders, & Street, 1988) were found. The reference lists of the reviews were examined for possible nurse authors. In spite of an extensive search, some authors may have been missed. Not all journals report the discipline of the authors, and not all nurses identify themselves. Furthermore, book chapters or articles in conference proceedings may have been missed. The chapter is organized according to historical perspective, review of the studies, and summary and directions for future research.

HISTORICAL PERSPECTIVE

Freud, in his 1917 paper "Mourning and Melancholia," defined mourning as a normal psychologic process occurring after the loss by death of an emotionally important person (p. 243). Research on children and death emerged in the 1940s when Anthony (1940) conducted a study on children's concept of death. Many studies on children's understanding of death followed (Childers & Wimmer, 1971; Koocher, 1974; Nagera, 1964; Nagy, 1948). Nurse researchers also conducted studies contributing to the understanding of children's concept of death (Swain, 1979; Waechter, 1971). Research on children's grief and mourning, however, did not begin until the early 1950s with a report by Bowlby (1960) in which he described a pattern of behavior, denial–protest–apathy, in young children when they were separated from their parents. Bowlby (1961, 1982) developed a theory of attachment and loss in which he hypothesized that the emotional distress of bereavement (grief and mourning) was the result of severing the bonds of attachment in highly valued relationships. Several authors contest the belief that children can and do grieve (Fleming & Altschul, 1963; Rochlin, 1965; Wolfenstein 1966, 1969). Although it is acknowledged that a distinct pattern of behavior emerges as a result of the loss, the incomplete development of ego function and dependence on significant others is believed to inhibit grief and mourning, and thus resolution of the loss (Miller, 1971). Furman (1974) proposed that children could be assisted in the grieving process by a supportive adult. The general belief is that the experience of bereavement for children is fraught with danger for their personality development, academic achievement, and psychologic well-being (Berlinsky & Biller, 1982; Masterman & Reams, 1988).

Berlinsky and Biller (1982) conducted an extensive review of the childhood bereavement literature. Several criticisms of the extant studies evolved from their review. Criticisms included: emphasis on parental loss and oversight of other more frequently occurring losses, such as siblings and grandparents; use of subjects seeking or referred for help; small and convenience samples; poorly designed studies lacking scientific rigor; and lack of theoretical bases to guide research.

Nursing research on childhood and adolescent bereavement followed in the wake of the controversy as to whether or not children can or do actually grieve. Nurse researchers have viewed childhood and adolescent bereavement from a variety of conceptual perspectives, for example, relationship to the deceased, parental support, parents' bereavement responses, location of the death (home or hospital), and impact on the child's development and self-concept.

Benoliel (1983) reviewed literature on death, dying, and terminal illness. Her review included an excellent historical perspective on the development of research related to the field of thanatology. In the historical perspective she outlined the work leading to conceptualization of grief and mourning in children. Benoliel's review included studies related to the nature and development of children's understanding of death, but did not include review of studies on childhood bereavement. Demi and Miles (1986) reviewed the bereavement literature and included a section on children's bereavement in which they reviewed three extant nursing studies (Long, 1983; Mandell, McAnulty, & Carlson, 1983; Mulhern, Lauer, & Hoffman, 1983). Betz (1987), in a review of the bereavement literature, categorized the literature as follows: (a) children's conception of death, (b) childhood bereavement responses, (c) research on responses of the dying child, and (d) parental response to loss of a child. Betz concluded that most nursing research on childhood bereavement was related to loss of a sibling.

Valente, Saunders, and Street (1988) examined the general field of research related to adolescent bereavement following the suicide of a parent, sibling, or peer. The authors concluded that the related research was very sparse and often marred by sampling bias and methodologic flaws. Recommendations made by the reviewers were consistent and similar to those made by reviewers of bereavement research in other disciplines. Recommendations included use of reliable and valid instruments; improved designs (qualitative, multivariate, and experimental) guided by conceptual or theoretical models; more representative and larger samples that include minorities, males, and lower-class persons; and clarification of the grief process from bereavement outcome.

REVIEW OF NURSING STUDIES

Eleven nursing studies focused on childhood and adolescent bereavement were reviewed, one of which was a report of instrument development (Hogan, 1990). The remainder of the studies investigated childhood and adolescent bereavement phenomena. Studies were critiqued for the focus and theoretical or conceptual basis; sample size and characteristics and sampling process; design and methodologic issues, findings, and conclusions; and the contribution to nursing knowledge. The review is organized by developmental level of the research samples, childhood, adolescent, and mixed age samples.

Childhood

Four studies were found investigating the bereavement phenomena of childhood (Carter, 1986a, 1986b; Long, 1983; Mandell et al., 1983; Mulhern et al., 1983). Long's report focused on the multitude of losses sustained by Crow Indian children and the behaviors exhibited in relating to the nurse therapist. Her report was descriptive, using two case studies to exemplify her descriptions of the children and the type and extent of their losses. The Crow Indian lifestyle, cultural beliefs, and behavioral prescriptions were described and used to explain the children's avoidance of feelings and passive behavior. No theoretical formulation was provided by the author. The design and methods for data gathering were not described, nor the number of children observed. The author described the children from the vantage point of therapist and consultant. Characteristics of the sample were provided in only a general sense and described in terms of types of losses, how the losses occurred (death, family description, clan rules, prescriptions), and generally how children related to the nurse therapist. While this article has multiple limitations, it was a seminal article in nursing on loss and bereavement in a specific childhood population.

Mandell et al. (1983) investigated behavioral change in preschool children after the loss of a sibling by Sudden Infant Death Syndrome (SIDS). A theoretical formulation was not provided for the study. Descriptions of behavior change in the area of parent–child interactions, sleeping, toileting and feeding behaviors, and peer social behavior were investigated for a convenience sample of 35 siblings in 26 families. Subjects ranged in age from 16 months to 6 years at the time of the sibling's death and were equally divided by sex. Families were described as being predominantly in the lower middle to upper lower class. The sample was limited to a Northeastern geographic area. The mother in each family was questioned using an interview schedule to obtain information about changes in the children's behavior. Interviews lasted 30 to 60 minutes, but the report does not indicate where the interview occurred. The interview schedule was not described (e.g., development strategy, content validity, number and type of items, response format, etc.) nor was information provided on data management. Findings were presented in frequencies and percentages. Separation anxiety was the most consistent child behavior change noted. Sleep disturbance (difficulty falling asleep) was the second most frequently reported behavioral change. Findings were attributed to loss of an anticipated role and parental behavioral changes. Conclusions derived by the authors included that physicians need to be more sensitive to the needs of the total family in SIDS. They suggested caution in generalizing the findings due to lack of a comparison group. In spite of a nursing co-author, implications for nursing were not provided. Utilization of a nonbereaved comparison group, standardization of the interview schedule, and content on data management would greatly improve confidence in the findings. The exploration of behavioral changes and needs in siblings and their families following a SIDS death was and continues to be a fertile area for study.

The third study in the childhood group (Mulhern et al., 1983) investigated behavioral changes in a convenience sample of children four to 13 years after the death of a sibling due to cancer. The sibling of 28 subjects had died at home (Home Care Group) and for 17 subjects, the sibling had died in the hospital (Hospital Care Group). Family socioeconomic status (SES) was measured by the Hollingshead Index. One-third of the families were classified as middle to upper class; the remainder were in the lower two classes. Behavior of the child subjects was measured using the Louisville Behavior Checklist (LBC) (Miller, 1977), a 164-item standardized inventory. Multivariate and univariate analyses were conducted. The Home Care Group compared favorably with normalized scores provided for the LBC, whereas the Hospital Care Group had scores on two subscales, Fear and Neuroticism, suggesting clinical significance. No differences were found between younger and older age groups. Confidence in the findings would have been strengthened by prospective evaluation of subjects before entry to the choice of program. A theoretical or conceptual framework was not identified in the report and implications for nursing were not addressed.

The descriptive study reported by Carter (1986) involved teachers' assessment of schoolaged children. Fourteen teachers responded to an 11-item, investigator-developed questionnaire. Content and face validity and response format were not described. The response rate of teachers was 66%. Percentages of children having lost a parent, grandparent, or sibling were reported, as well as behavioral changes. However, the actual number of children in question, their ages, socioeconomic status, or other characteristics were not reported. Data management (content analysis of responses) and statistical analysis were not described and no theoretical or conceptual framework was provided. The author does not explain her findings. She does suggest that nurses should work more closely with teachers to provide support for teachers and the bereaved children. The sample design, methods, and instrumentation for this study should have been described in more depth.

Adolescence

Three studies were found that focused on adolescent bereavement issues and that used only adolescent subjects. The three studies were authored or co-authored by Hogan (1988); Hogan and Balk (1990); and Hogan (1990). The last study addressed instrument development.

In the first study, Hogan (1988) investigated the concept of time since loss and its relationship to grief and mourning behaviors in adolescents. This descriptive correlational study utilized a convenience sample of 40 thirteen- to eighteen-year-old adolescents who had experienced the death of a sibling due to illness, accident, or suicide. Subjects were largely white (82%), Catholic (62%), Midwestern, and involved in a mutual-help organization. The 109-item, investigator-developed instrument (Hogan Sibling Inventory of Bereavement, HSIB) was used to measure the grief response. A reliability coefficient of .88 was reported. Time since the death was categorized as the first 18 months and the second 18 months. Findings during the first 18 months included assignment of blame to self and difficulty sleeping and concentrating. During the second 18 months subjects significantly more often reported attribution of blame to God and reported a sense of the family being "normal again." Findings were discussed in terms of implications for the academic setting, for parents, and for nursing practice. This study could have been improved by utilizing a random sample and a comparison group of teenagers who were not involved in a support group. The moderate size of the sample, reliability of the instrument, and concept-driven nature of the study are noteworthy.

Hogan and Balk (1990) investigated parent and subject ratings of self-concept of 13- to 18-year-old adolescents after loss of a sibling. The sample of 14 (7 boys, 7 girls) was obtained from a mutual-help group. Seventy-six percent were white, 12% Hispanic, and 12% other racial identity. Twenty-eight parents (both parents of the subject) also rated the self-concept of their child, via utilization of the HSIB. Response format and reliability coefficients of .88 and .95 were reported. The investigators found that father's ratings of the adolescent's self-concept was more closely related to the ratings reported by the adolescent subjects, than the rating given by mothers. The authors contrasted their findings with other research findings and noted the need for health care professionals to be aware of complex family dynamics in the grief and mourning process. Comparing and relating the findings of this analysis to that of the 1988 study by Hogan would have enhanced the ability to draw implications from the study findings.

Hogan (1990) reported on the development of an instrument to measure adolescent bereavement, the Hogan Sibling Inventory of Bereavement (HSIB). The 109-item, self-report inventory has a 5-point response scale ranging from 1 (almost always true) to 5 (hardly ever true). The instrument can be used as a whole or divided into five subscales (peer relations, family, school, self-concept, and grief reactions). The items evolved from an extensive review of literature and discussion with adolescent bereavement experts. One hundred forty-four adolescents participated in the testing of the instrument. Internal consistency for the total scale ranged from .73 to .95.

Mixed Ages

Four studies used children and adolescents as subjects. Demi and Gilbert (1987) investigated the correlation of parental emotional distress, grief patterns, and role dysfunction with the responses of their children's degree of emotional distress, grief patterns, and behavior problems after death of a child (sibling). Bowen's family systems theory provided direction for this investigation. The sample, 22 parent–child pairs (14 parents and 18 siblings) was obtained through professional contacts with known subjects and names obtained from vital statistics records. The majority of subjects were white and from the lower socioeconomic class. A structured interview was used to obtain descriptive characteristics. Three instruments [Impact of Events Scale (IES) (Horowitz, Wilner, Alverez, 1979), Child Depression Inventory (Kovacs & Beck, 1977), and the Child Behavior Checklist (Achenbach & Edelbrock, 1979)] with established reliability were used to measure emotional distress, grief patterns, and behavior of child subjects. The IES, Hopkins Symptoms Checklist (Derogatis, Lipman, Rickels, Uhlen, & Covi, 1974), and the Parental Role Scale (Weisman & Bothwell, 1977) were used to measure parental grieving and parental role functioning. The Pearson correlation was used to test hypotheses. A significant positive correlation was found between parental emotional distress and the child's emotional distress, and between parental role dysfunction and child behavior problems. A direct positive relationship was found between child avoidance scores and parent grief pattern of intrusion. Parents scored higher on intrusive thoughts, whereas children scored higher on avoidance and denial. The authors discussed their findings in relation to developmental theory, previous research, and to Bowen's (1978) family systems theory. Limitations of the study addressed by the investigators were the small and nonrandom sample, and the data collection at only one time in the bereavement process. Implications for practice were generalized to all health care providers. As noted by the authors, the study would have been improved by increasing the sample size. The careful attention to development of hypotheses derived from a theoretical framework and multivariate nature of the investigation were notable strengths of the study.

Martinson, Davies, and McClowery (1987) and McClowery, Davies, May, Kulenkamp, and Martinson (1987) reported on different aspects of the same study. Interviews were conducted with 58 families, 7 to 9 years after the death of a child who had been involved in a home health program. Twenty-nine siblings (9 to 18 years) completed the Piers-Harris Self-Concept Scale (Martinson et al., 1987). Their subjects scored higher than the normative sample. The authors concluded that the experience with death and subsequent coping may have produced greater maturity and respect for the self. McClowery et al. (1987) used the interview data to describe patterns of family management of the "empty space" caused by the loss. Subjects' responses were included in family responses to describe three resolution patterns that emerged from the data. McClowery et al. (1987) used a semistructured interview and 9 grounded theory approach to analyze the data. Development of and the source of interview schedule items was not provided. Martinson et al. and McClowery et al. provided implications for practice and noted that the subjects had received special help at the time of the loss. The sample size was adequate for the two analyses; however, the study could have been improved by utilization of a comparison group that had received no home care or hospitalization.

Davies (1988) investigated the concept of "closeness" (operationalized as shared life space) and sibling bereavement responses. Attachment theory provided direction for the development of the study. Fifty-five subjects, 6 to 16 years old, were obtained from pediatric clinics and a mutual-help organization. All were white, Protestant, and middle class. Instruments used were the Closeness Index (CI) developed by the investigator, the Child Behavior Checklist (CBCL) (Achenbach & Edelbrock, 1977), and an investigator-developed interview schedule. Reliabilities for the CI and CBCL were reported. Content validity was established for the interview schedule. The correlation between bereavement outcome (CBCL) and closeness (CI) was not significant. However, closeness was correlated with internalizing behavior scores. Limitations noted by the author were the nonprobability sample, use of parental report data collected during a stressful period for the parent, and lack of generalizability to ethnic families and nonmiddle class SES groups. Implications for nursing practice and recommendations for future research were provided.

SUMMARY

Theoretical/Conceptual Bases

A theoretical or conceptual focus directed study development and interpretation of findings in eight of the 11 studies reviewed. Concepts of affective bonds (shared space, empty space), time since loss, and self-concept were derived from the bereavement literature and previous related research. One study (Demi & Gilbert, 1987) derived concepts and hypotheses from a family systems theory frequently used by nurses. Another study (Hogan & Balk, 1990) used an eclectic approach to development of their conceptual framework. Literature that guided development of the Hogan and Balk study was previous research by the authors, social support, and family stress and coping literature. Utilization of nursing theory was not evidenced in any of the studies.

Most authors stated implications as being relevant to health care providers generally. Most authors did not relate implications of their findings directly to nursing theory or practice. The three studies lacking a theoretical or conceptual basis (Carter 1986; Long 1983; Mandell et al., 1983) addressed populations with special needs and raised important issues for nurses to address in future studies. Carter's study raises questions about children's academic functioning and emotional well-being after the loss of grandparents and the role of the school nurse in assisting teachers to cope with bereaved children in the academic setting. Long's study raises important questions about the relationship of bereavement outcomes to concurrent stressors such as poverty, cultural variable, nontraditional family styles, and multiple losses. Mandell et al. introduced the concept of loss of an anticipated role or new role for preschool children when a SIDS death occurs in a family.

Hogan (1988, 1990; Hogan & Balk, 1990) is the only author who demonstrated development of a "line of inquiry." Her work includes instrument development and follow-up studies to test the instrument and the concepts addressed in the instrument. Hogan's research (conceptual and instrument development) represents seminal work in the adolescent nursing bereavement literature.

Sampling

A major criticism of the child and adolescent bereavement literature has been that significant losses, other than parent loss, were overlooked or ignored. Nurse researchers have, on the other hand, focused almost exclusively on sibling loss. Nine of the 11 studies were related to loss of a sibling. Four of the studies involved sibling death due to cancer, and three of these studies involved samples that had been involved in special care programs. Four studies used sibling samples where the cause of death was varied. However, in three studies subjects were drawn from a mutual-help support group. Mulhern et al. (1983), using mutual-help support group members, provided the only comparison sample among the studies. Long (1983) and Carter (1986) provided the only studies that did not focus exclusively on sibling loss. Unfortunately, the lack of scientific rigor of the latter two studies limited the contribution to the body of knowledge on childhood bereavement.

Three studies were focused exclusively on adolescent bereavement phenomena, one of which addressed instrument development. Adolescent subjects were included in four studies using mixed-age samples. It can be said that nurse researchers are aware of needs across the developmental span of childhood; however, there is a need to direct more research toward the study of bereavement phenomena in the preschool years.

Nurse researchers included subjects from the lower SES groups in 10 studies; however, examination of the samples demonstrates a significant lack of ethnic and minority variability among the subjects. In one study 11% of the sample was Hispanic. Generally, the samples were white and lower to middle class. Due to the small number of studies and the frequent sampling bias, it can be concluded that no single population has been adequately studied.

Design and Methodologic Issues

Three studies used a single sample descriptive design and lacked a conceptual focus beyond behavior change and problems occurring after loss. In one study (Mandell et al., 1983) the descriptive statistics used to present the findings were appropriate to the design; however, there is no description of type of data obtained, and thus the findings and conclusions may be questioned. The second study (Carter, 1986) also presented findings in percentages; however, there was sufficient lack of clarity regarding her data and methods that confidence could not be placed in the findings. Long (1983) used a case study (descriptive) approach; thus, no statistical analysis was provided.

Authors of three studies (Martinson et al., 1987; McClowery et al., 1987; Mulhern et al., 1983) used ex post facto designs; one of these (Mulhern et al., 1983) used a comparison group. This was the only study to use this methodologic control. Of this group of studies, both Martinson et al. and Mulhern et al., used standardized, reliable instruments and inferential statistics. Martinson et al. (1987) compared their findings to the normed scores for the instrument. McClowery et al. (1987) used interview data and appropriately a grounded theory approach (content and latent analysis) to manage the nominal data. Four studies (Davies, 1988; Demi & Gilbert, 1987; Hogan, 1988; Hogan & Balk, 1990) used correlational designs and inferential statistics (Pearson correlation, *t*-tests, and regression analysis) appropriate to the design and type of data. The final study (Hogan, 1990) was a methodologic study that focused on instrument development.

The study designs continue to contain flaws that have plagued the child bereavement research. Surprisingly, only two authors (Davies, 1988; Demi & Gilbert, 1987) acknowledged the limitations inherent in their studies. Limitations included small, nonrepresentative samples, lack of comparison groups, and unclear definitions of the research focus, for example, grief process versus bereavement outcome. In several studies, instrumentation and description of data collection procedures and data management were inadequate.

Findings and Conclusions

Findings may be categorized as positive, negative, mixed, and factors influencing bereavement outcome or process. Carter (1986), Long (1983), and Mandell et al. (1983) all reported that the experience of bereavement produced negative consequences, for example, behavioral changes, (Mandell et al., 1983), emotional flattening and interpersonal distancing (Long, 1983), or academic problems (Carter, 1986). The authors attributed their findings to the experience of loss of a loved one (Carter, 1987) or anticipated role (Mandell, 1983). Long (1983) attributed her observations to the interplay of multiple losses, concurrent stressors, and cultural variables.

Positive findings were reported on self-concept and behavioral measures by Martinson et al. (1987) and Mulhern et al. (1983). Subjects in the two studies had been involved in a special program for dying children at the time of the sibling death. Subjects in the Mulhern et al. study were surveyed 3 to 19 months after the sibling death. Martinson et al. surveyed subjects 7 to 9 years after the sibling death. Mulhern et al. concluded that children in the Home Care Program were adjusting significantly better than the comparison group, whose sibling had died in the hospital. Martinson et al. concluded that the Home Care Program was conducive to long-term positive outcomes for bereaved siblings. Hogan and Balk (1990) also reported positive bereavement outcomes for their subjects.

Mixed findings were reported by McClowery et al. (1987) on family adjustment to a sibling death. Family management of the empty space was categorized, suggesting two methods providing resolution of grief and a third suggesting continued focus on loss and emotional distress.

Four studies (Davies, 1988; Demi & Gilbert, 1987; Hogan, 1988; Hogan & Balk, 1990) provided findings related to factors influencing the process and/or outcome of bereavement. Factors found to be correlated ith the process and intensity of the sibling's grief were degree of parental distress and function (Demi & Gilbert, 1987), the affective bond between the deceased and surviving sibling (Davis, 1988), and time since the death with subjects in the second 18 months of bereavement demonstrating greater resolution of the loss (Hogan, 1988). The Hogan and Balk (1990) study suggested that fathers, although perceived as less involved in their child's grief process, had a more accurate view of the child's resolution state and self-concept than did mothers.

DIRECTIONS FOR FUTURE RESEARCH

The findings raise varied but important questions that need to be addressed in future research. The limitations inherent in the research support the need for studies with improved designs and more representative samples, in addition to studies that investigate new and different questions, for example, the effect of multiple stressors, bereavement rituals and processes in varied cultural and ethnic groups, and intervention studies, to mention a few. Childhood and adolescent bereavement is a rich and fertile area in which many questions can be raised for investigation, but nurse researchers would do well to conduct repeated studies, especially when small sample sizes are necessary and other limitations cannot be rectified. Rigorously designed qualitative and multivariate studies would enhance this field of research.

In several of the studies, researchers used interview schedules that were not fully described in terms of content validity or development. Structured interview schedules and questionnaires need to be developed systematically, based on literature reviews and consultation with experts when appropriate. Content validity, construct validity, and stability of the instruments needs to be extended and improved for descriptive studies. Davies (1988) and Hogan (1990) made important contributions in the development of new instruments. Studies published after 1986 show improvement in the utilization of standardized and reliable instruments and in clarity of the concepts being tested.

Little is known about the effect of interventions for bereaved children and adolescents. Some nurse researchers refuted the often touted poor outcome for bereaved children and adolescents. Factors influencing this more positive outlook may be due to the type of loss (sibling versus parent) investigated and the sample source (groups who had received special attention during the terminal state of the sibling's illness or were receiving some assistance and support at the time of data collection). The findings provided in studies with samples that have received or are receiving special recognition or help are provocative, but without comparison groups and studies designed specifically to test interventions, nursing's knowledge is incomplete. Owing to the high-risk nature of the bereaved child and adolescent population the development of programs of intervention research with control groups is of utmost importance. Research is needed to determine the best interventions and for which populations they are effective. Knowledge of the appropriate time to offer interventions and the needed length and intensity of interventions is also much needed. Review of nonnursing bereavement research with children demonstrates that intervention research has been overlooked in other disciplines as well as nursing (Masterman & Reams, 1988)

Nurses have raised important theoretical considerations and have investigated some very relevant concepts. However, without continued systematic research to further test and explicate the conceptual relationships underlying childhood and adolescent bereavement, theory development cannot take place. Development of a program of research to test concepts with a variety of subjects and to measure the relationship of concepts to one another is a necessary step in the development of theory.

This review demonstrated a continued involvement of nurses in childhood bereavement research. Progress has occurred in the utilization of theoretical and conceptual frameworks to guide study development and discussion of findings. Some work has occurred on development of reliable instruments based on concepts related and important to childhood and adolescent bereavement. Nurse researchers have recognized sibling death as a significant loss for children and adolescents and have concentrated their research endeavors on this previously neglected topic. Although progress has occurred, this review provides direction for improvement and expansion of future research.

REFERENCES

Achenbach, T. M. (1979). The child behavior profile: An empirically based system for assessing children's behavioral problems and competencies. *International Journal of Mental Health, 4,* 24–42.

Achenbach, T. M., & Edelbrock, C. (1979). The child behavior profile: II. Boys aged 12–16 and girls aged 6–11 and 12–16. *Journal Consulting & Clinical Psychology, 47,* 223–233.
Anthony, S. (1940). *The child's discovery of death.* New York: Harcourt.
Benoliel, J. Q. (1984). Nursing research on death, dying and terminal illness: Development, present state and prospects. In H. H. Werley & J. J. Fitzpatrick (Eds.), *Annual review of nursing research* (pp. 101–130). New York: Springer Publishing Co.
Berlinsky, E., & Biller, H. (1982). *Parental death and psychological development.* Lexington, MA: Lexington Books.
Betz, C. L. (1987). Death, dying, and bereavement: A review of the literature, 1970–1985. In T. Krulick, B. Holaday, & I. M. Martinson (Eds.), *The child and family facing life-threatening illness* (pp. 39–49). Philadelphia: Lippincott.
Bowen, M. (1978). *Family therapy and clinical practice.* Northvale, NJ: Jason Aronson.
Bowlby, J. (1960). Grief and mourning in infancy and early childhood. *Psychoanalytic Study of the Child, 15,* 9–52.
Bowlby, J. (1961). Childhood mourning and its implications for psychiatry. *American Journal of Psychiatry, 118,* 481–498.
Bowlby, J. (1982). Attachment and loss: Retrospect and prospect. *The American Journal of Orthopsychiatry, 52,* 664–678.
Carter, P. (1986a). School nursing: Helping children to grieve. *Community Outlook,* August, 16–17 (Part I).
Carter, P. (1986b). School nursing: Helping children to grieve. *Community Outlook, September,* 16–20 (Part II).
Childers, P., & Wimmer, M. (1971). The concept of death in early childhood. *Child Development, 42,* 1299–1301.
Davies, B. (1988). Shared life space and sibling bereavement responses. *Cancer Nursing, 11,* 339–347.
Demi, A. S., & Gilbert, C. M. (1987). Relationship of parental grief to sibling grief. *Archives of Psychiatric Nursing, 1,* 385–391.
Demi, A. S., & Miles, M. S. (1986). Bereavement. In H. H. Werley, J. J. Fitzpatrick, & R. L. Taunton (Eds.), *Annual review of nursing research,* Volume 6 (pp. 105–123). New York: Springer Publishing Co.
Derogatis, L. R., Lipman, R. S., Rickels, K., Uhlenhuth, E. H., & Covi, L. (1974). The Hopkins Symptom Checklist (HSCL): A self report symptom inventory. *Behavioral Science, 19*(1), 1–15.
Fleming, J., & Altschul, S. (1963). Activation of mourning and growth by psychoanalysis. *International Journal of Psychoanalysis, 44,* 419–432.
Freud, S. (1957 original work published in 1917). Mourning and Melancholia. In J. Strachey (Ed. & Trans.), *The Standard edition of the complete psychological works of Sigmund Freud.* (Vol. 14) (pp. 243–258). London: Hogarth Press.
Furman, E. (1974). *A child's parent dies.* New Haven, CT: Yale University Press.
Hogan, N. S. (1988). The effects of time on the adolescent sibling bereavement process. *Pediatric Nursing, 14,* 333–335.
Hogan, N. S. (1990). Hogan Sibling Inventory of Bereavement. In J. Touriatos, B. Perlmutter, & M. Strauss (Eds.), *Handbook of family measurement techniques* (p. 524). Newbury Park, CA: Sage.
Hogan, N. S., & Balk, D. E. (1990). Adolescent reactions to sibling death: Perceptions of mothers, fathers and teenagers. *Nursing Research, 39,* 103–106.

Horowitz, M., Wilner, N., & Alverez, W. (1979). Impact of Event Scale: A measure of subjective distress. *Psychosomatic Medicine, 41,* 209–218.
Koocher, G. (1974). Talking with children about death. *American Journal of Orthopsychiatry, 44,* 404–411.
Kovacs, M., & Beck, A. (1977). An empirical-clinical approach toward a definition of childhood depression. In J. Schulterbrandt & A. Raskin, (Eds.), *Depression in childhood: Diagnosis, treatment, and conceptual models* (pp. 1–25). New York: Raven Press.
Long, K. A. (1983). The experience of repeated and traumatic loss among Crow Indian children: Response patterns and intervention strategies. *American Journal of Orthopsychiatry, 53,* 116–126.
Mandell, F., McAnulty, E., & Carlson, A. (1983). Unexpected death of an infant sibling. *Pediatrics, 72,* 652–657.
Martinson, I. M., Davies, E. B., & McClowery, S. G. (1987). The long-term effects of sibling death on self-concept. *Journal of Pediatric Nursing, 2,* 227–235.
Masterman, S. H., & Reams, R. (1988). Support groups for bereaved pre-school and school-aged children. *American Journal of Orthopsychiatry, 58,* 562–570.
McClowery, S. G., Davies, E. B., May, K. A., Kulenkamp, E. J., & Martinson, I. M. (1987). The empty space phenomenon: The process of grief in the bereaved family. *Death Studies, 11,* 361–374.
Miller, J. B. (1971). Reactions to the death of a parent: A review of psychoanalytical literature. *American Psychoanalysis Association, 19,* 697–719.
Miller, L. C. (1977). *Louisville Behavior Checklist Manual.* Los Angeles: Western Psychological Services.
Mulhern, R. K., Lauer, M. E., & Hoffman, R. G. (1983). Death of a child at home or in the hospital: Subsequent psychological adjustment of the family. *Pediatrics, 71,* 743–747.
Nagera, H. (1964). Children's reactions to the death of important objects. *Psychoanalytic Study of the Child, 19,* 360–400.
Nagy, M. (1948). The child's theories concerning death. *Journal of Genetic Psychology, 73,* 3–27.
Piers, E. (1976). *The Piers-Harris Self-Concept Scale.* (Research monograph no. 1). Nashville, TN: Counselor Recordings and Tests.
Rochlin, G. (1965). *Grief and discontents.* Boston: Little, Brown.
Swain, H. L. (1979). Childhood views of death. *Death Education, 2,* 341–358.
Valente, S., Saunders, J., & Street, R. (1988). Adolescent bereavement following suicide: An examination of relevant literature. *Journal of Counseling and Development, 67,* 174–177.
Waechter, E. H. (1971). Children's awareness of fatal illness. *American Journal of Nursing, 71,* 1168–1172.
Weissman, M. M., & Bothwell, S. (1977). *The assessment of social adjustment by patient self-report.* Unpublished manuscript.
Wolfenstein, M. (1966). How is mourning possible? (Ed.), *The Psychoanalytic Study of the Child, 21,* 93–123.
Wolfenstein, M. (1969). Loss, rage, and repetition. *The Psychoanalytic Study of the Child, 24,* 432–460.

PART II

Research on Nursing Care Delivery

Chapter 8

Nursing Centers

SUSAN K. RIESCH
SCHOOL OF NURSING
UNIVERSITY OF WISCONSIN-MILWAUKEE

CONTENTS

A nursing center is both a setting and a concept. Other names used synonymously with nursing center are nurse-managed center, community nursing center or organization, or nurse-run clinic. An analysis of the extensive anecdotal and the limited empirical literature on nursing centers led to the conclusion that nursing center leaders have made substantial contributions to the definition and refinement of nursing practice, but the research base needs considerable development.

The extensive anecdotal literature contained many definitions of nursing centers. The dominant themes gleaned were that practice and patient care are directly accessible by patients/clients, are nurse controlled, and serve to shape future generations of nurses. Since 1982 biennial national conferences have been held to promote networking among nurses affiliated with nursing centers*. In 1984, a modified Delphi survey method was used with a sample of

*A compilation of conference-sponsoring institutions, agendas, and abstracts is available from the author.

143 nurses, chiefly master's prepared practitioners and educators attending the Second Biennial Conference on Nursing Centers. The Delphi questionnaire was developed by Fehring, Schulte, and Riesch (1987) to reflect the issues found in the literature such as practice models, administration, and cost of nursing centers. After three rounds of data collection, the following definition resulted:

> Nursing centers are organizations that provide direct access to professional nurses who offer holistic client-centered health services for reimbursement. With the use of nursing models of health, professional nurses in nursing centers diagnose and treat human responses to potential and actual health problems. Examples of professional nursing services include health education, health promotion, and health-related research. Services are targeted to individuals and groups whose health needs are not being met (e.g., the poor, women, elderly, minorities) by current systems. An effective referral system and collaboration with other health care professionals are an integral part of nursing centers. As models of professional nursing practice and research, nursing centers are ideal sites for a faculty and student practice. They are administered by a professional nurse. (p. 63)

Limitations of this study were that the survey instrument was not developed by the expert sample as the Delphi Technique requires, all three rounds occurred in 2 days, and only experts in attendance at the conference were included in the sample. However, the investigators obtained a beginning consensus on the chief concepts of a nursing center. This definition is referred to frequently in the literature (Bagwell, 1987; Barger, 1987; Burgess, 1988).

This review was limited to an analysis of the empirical literature. To compile research on nursing centers, the Bibliographic Retrieval Services (BRS) Information Technologies computerized system was used to search the literature from 1979 to 1989. The key words were nursing center, nursing clinic, nurse managed/run center/clinic, and community nursing organization. In addition, the abstracts from all four national biennial conferences on nursing centers were reviewed. Theses and dissertations about nursing centers were not included.

HISTORICAL REVIEW

Nurses have struggled to define and control their practice as well as "separate clearly the medical and nursing provinces" (Dock, 1949) since Nightingale's time. In a provocative paper presented at the Fourth Biennial Conference on Nursing Centers, Glass (1988) asserted that visiting nursing, also called district nursing, eventually gave way to public health nursing, which in turn led to the concept of nursing centers. Visiting nursing, Glass stated, had its origins in the resurgence of humanitarianism that occurred at the end of the 19th century. Visiting nurses first were sent out in 1877 by the Women's Branch of the New York City Mission, followed by the Boston Instructive Nursing Association in 1886 and the Chicago Hull House in 1889.

The New York Henry Street Settlement House, founded by Lillian Wald and Mary Brewster in 1893, became the New York Visiting Nurses Association. This practice was based on Wald's notion that nurses should be at the "call of the people who need them without intervention of a medical man" (Woolf, 1937). Margaret Sanger, working at the Henry Street Settlement, is credited with the national family planning movement. She advocated women's control over their reproductive health. In 1916 she developed the first birth control clinic in the world—other than those in the Netherlands (Sanger, 1971)

In 1925, Mary Breckenridge founded the Frontier Nursing Service to provide health and midwifery services to mothers and infants. There were six decentralized nursing centers: all were named for donors; each center served a 5-mile radius. These centers were supported by a prospective payment system in which "subscriptions of not less than a dollar from every householder" once a year were "payable in money or in kind" (Resolutions, 1925). This service has retained its original philosophy today (Burgess, 1988).

According to Glass (1988), these centers were the result of strong, impassioned leadership. They were dedicated to providing nursing care and teaching to poor and needy persons as well as to serving as nurse training sites.

Creative sources of funding, such as the Red Cross and Metropolitan Life Insurance Company, were tapped. However, income was not a motivating factor to the clinic developers. In fact, the New York Visiting Nurses Association and Metropolitan Life Insurance Company disbanded because the insurance company thought the Visiting Nurses Association did not have enough concern for the economic aspects of practice.

CONTEMPORARY RESURGENCE

The literature is devoid of reports of nursing center development until the 1960s. In 1963 Lydia Hall established the nurse-managed Loeb Center in New York. Hall (1963) wrote that the Loeb Center was a "nursing center with an organization of service and programs . . . close to public health nursing . . . in an institutional setting" (p. 805).

Milio (1970), Kinlein (1972), and Henry (1978) espoused the concept that new knowledge could be developed from experience in practice. Although they were not writing specifically about nursing centers, the nursing practices established by them had characteristics similar to those of nursing centers. Major ideas underlying these writings were that nursing: (a) is not under the supervision of other disciplines but delineates its own scope of practice; (b) is accountable and responsible for patient, family, and community care 24 hours per day, seven days per week; and (c) is responsible for socializing its students and practitioners in practice, research, and administration.

During the 1970s and 1980s, a resurgence of nursing centers occurred that can be traced to two factors. The first was the paucity of clinical teaching sites with well populations for undergraduate and graduate student experiences (Arlton & Miercort, 1980; Barger, 1986a; Chickadonz, Burke, Fitzgerald, & Osterweis, 1982; Higgs, 1985; Mezey & Chiamulera, 1980; Ossler, Goodwin, Mariani, & Gilliss, 1982; Riesch, Felder, & Stauder, 1980). The second was increased opportunities to develop demonstration projects or research environments with underserved populations (Baird & Benner, 1985; Hawkins, Igou, Johnson, & Utley, 1984; Hill, 1986; Kogan, et al., 1983; Thibodeau & Hawkins, 1987). The nursing center resurgence was assisted greatly by a series of initiatives from federal and state legislatures, private foundations, and professional organizations.

STATE OF THE ART OF RESEARCH ON NURSING CENTERS

According to a survey by Riesch, Fehring, Schulte, and Wright (1986), little research has been conducted in nursing centers, despite a reflection of this activity in most center philosophies. The convenience sample for the study consisted of any center representative who contacted the Nursing Center at the University of Wisconsin-Milwaukee for information regarding nursing centers ($n = 50$). The dearth of research conducted was attributed to fiscal vulnerability, lack of research trained staff, and an identification of clinical practice as the primary focus of nursing centers. Notwithstanding, respondents to the survey indicated that they based care protocols on current research and encouraged nursing faculty and students to conduct research at the center.

In addition to the definition of a center, to date researchers have addressed the location and demographic profiles of academic centers; student outcomes; client and patient outcomes such as knowledge, attitude, behavior, health status, and satisfaction with care; and cost effectiveness and quality of care.

Location and Demographic Profile of Nursing Centers

Barger (1986b) surveyed 427 National League for Nursing (NLN) accredited schools of nursing. Of 331 respondents, 51 reported having a nursing center. Barger found that most schools of nursing with nursing centers were not associated with an academic health science center or hospital, tended to have more than 35 faculty members, and junior and senior student enrollments greater than 200. Two-thirds had master's programs and one-fifth had doctoral programs. Barger found that faculties with nursing centers were more likely to consider faculty practice in workload and promotion decisions than faculties without a nursing center. However, schools with nursing centers did not require faculty practice, consider it in tenure decisions, or calculate the number of faculty positions based on it to any greater degree than faculty without a nursing center. Barger's (1986b) survey was limited to academic-based nursing centers. No systematic study of freestanding nursing centers was located.

Student Outcomes

Hauf (1977) studied outcomes of student experiences in an academic nursing center. The Nursing Services Center at Montana State University was the site for undergraduate students of community health nursing. Student activities included teaching prenatal classes, leading discussion groups on health-related topics, conducting health assessment and screening and developing community activities such as a multiple sclerosis chapter.

Data were gathered to determine if students from the nursing center site achieved the course objectives to the same degree as students in traditional site practicums.The sample included 24 students who were randomly selected from the senior class and assigned to the nursing center over a period of two university quarters. Learning outcomes were measured using teacher-made tests, a standardized achievement examination, preceptor evaluation, student self-evaluation, and course grade. A comparison group of students was selected from those having field experiences in public health agencies throughout the state. Groups were matched for age, grade-point average, and community health theory grade.

Using a Student's *t*-test to compare the two groups, Hauf (1977) found no differences between groups on any of the five measures. She concluded that variation in setting and activities did not influence learning community health nursing principles, but that the principles can be learned in alternative settings. Hauf did not present details about the instruments, sample characteristics, or activities of the traditional public health agency, nor was the data analysis sophisticated. The research was the only of its kind found in the literature.

Client Knowledge, Attitudes, and Behavior

The Nursing Center for Family Health Services was a joint venture of the Adelphi University School of Nursing and the Molloy College Department of Nursing. The Center functioned from 1972 to 1977 and provided service to low-income families in a geographically isolated housing project in surburban Long Island, New York. Kos and Rothberg (1981) evaluated the health knowledge, attitudes, and behavior of clients at this nursing center.

The sample consisted of 62 active, self-selected, adult clients of the Center who were between the ages of 16 and 77 years. The majority were female. The measurement instruments included two paper and pencil questionnaires and a structured interview schedule. The Attitudes toward Health–Student Health Services Scale [Woog et al. (study) cited in Kos & Rothberg, 1981] is a 20 item scale with a 5-point Likert-type format designed to measure satisfaction with personnel and health care provided. Ware's Behavioral Intention Scale [Ware (instrument) cited in Kos & Rothberg, 1981] lists six medical symptoms, some relatively serious and some not, to which the subject responded with one of eight possible actions to take upon discovery of such symptoms. The interview schedule was the Family Health Services Questionnaire that includes 13 interview items to assess the accuracy of patients' perceptions of their own health, the appropriateness of their health actions, their compliance with immunization schedules, and their definitions of what constitutes good health. No psychometric data were reported on any of the instruments, nor was the source of the Family Health Services Questionnaire identified.

Kos and Rothberg (1981) reported that their clients were satisfied with the care. Clients intended to use health professionals appropriately; that is, to limit seeking professional help to serious symptoms. A higher percentage (2 to 37%) of Kos and Rothberg's clients indicated that they intended to seek the services of nurses than did the project clients who served as subjects in the test development sample (1 to 5%). From these findings, Kos and Rothberg concluded that their clients had health knowledge and a high reliance on and comfort with the nurses and center as a primary source of health care.

Findings from the perceptions interview were inconsistent with the literature regarding health perceptions of low income populations. Kos and Rothberg (1981) reported that, for the most part, their sample's health perceptions were congruent with those of the nurse and were future or prevention oriented. Their use of medical resources was appropriate, and their immunization compliance was 83%. Definitions of health were not limited to the absence of disease but included physical and emotional well-being.

In a descriptive study of a nurse clinic run by a school of nursing, Muhlenkamp, Brown, and Sands (1985) administered questionnaires to the clients of the Community Health Services Clinic at Arizona State University to determine their health beliefs, values, and demographic characteristics. The 175 study participants were predominantly female, married, Caucasian protestants with a mean age of 28 years, less than a high school education, and an annual income of less than $10,000. Most described their health as good and made fewer than four visits to a health care provider per year.

The sample represented about 20% of the clinic caseload. The subjects completed well-established instruments to measure health locus-of-control (Wallston & Wallston, 1981), health values (Kaplan & Cowles, 1978), and personal lifestyle practices (Brown, Muhlenkamp, Fox & Osborn, 1983). The investigators approached the clients as they waited for their services at the clinic. The type of health care activity requested by the subject was obtained from the clinic record and coded as health promotion, illness prevention, health maintenance, or health restoration. The criteria for this coding were not described.

Muhlenkamp et al. (1985) determined that: (a) health values were not related to self-reported health promotion activities or types of clinic visits, (b) a strong belief in chance was negatively correlated with engaging in health promotion activities, and (c) a strong belief in powerful others was negatively associated with a high precentage of restoration visits. The combination of beliefs, values, and selected demographic factors accounted for 16% of the variance in health promotion activities and 18% of the variance in type of health care sought. Findings were interpreted with caution because the sample was highly internally controlled as measured by the locus-of-control scales. This study contributed to further evaluation and study of the Health Belief Model and added to the knowledge base of client attitudes and behaviors.

Using a quasi-experimental design, Duffy and Halloran (1987) developed and tested the effectiveness of a comprehensive supportive educational program offered at the University of Wisconsin-Milwaukee Nursing Center for parents of children with asthma. They measured parental knowledge and perceptions about their understanding, ability to deal with, and attitude toward asthma as well as parental perceptions of their child's understanding, ability to deal with, and attitude toward asthma before and after the program. The instruments developed for the study were understood clearly by the parents.

The majority of the sample (N = 35) were married women, high-school educated, in their early 30s, who had two children. Compared with their responses before the program, the investigators found a significant increase on all measures after the program except the parent's perception of the child's ability to deal with asthma. The authors concluded that group teaching modalities not only were effective cognitively and perceptually, but more cost effective than individual teaching. They recommended further study regarding long-term treatment effects, introduction of control conditions, and assessment of behavior change as a possible effect of the knowledge and perceptual changes.

Munroe and Natale (1982) analyzed after-hours calls to the Primary Care Nursing Service, a nurse faculty group delivering primary care to 1500 clients. Over an 18-month period (1978 to 1980), a total of 455 calls were recorded. Of these, 10% were administrative, 2% were iatrogenically induced concerns, and 20% were requests for information. Further study was done of the remaining 67% (N = 362) of the calls, which were considered to be requests for intervention. The top seven requests for intervention were for pain, gastrointestinal disturbance, bleeding, reproductive concern, need for prescription refill, respiratory dysfunction, and genitourinary disturbance. The interventions recorded were comfort, supportive measures, and reassurance; instruction to call the office; medication; status check; health information; referral to emergency room, other service, or physician; or instruction to discontinue or decrease medication.

From their data, the authors (Munroe & Natale, 1982) concluded that an after-hours call service is essential for a group primary care nursing practice. Patients usually expressed psychosocial or episodic needs and the dominant interventions were within the domain of nursing practice. The authors concluded that the after-hours call service was a method to reduce fragmentation of nursing practice for clients. The nurses who answered the after-hours calls were all master's prepared, experienced clinicians. Other than reporting that the clientele were mainly female between the ages of 14 and 90, there was little description of the sample from which the data were collected. Further, the outcomes of the phone intervention were not reported. This study, however, contributed to the definition of what nurses do and the services they provide.

Considered together, these studies on client knowledge, attitude, and behavior provide information about client needs, effective interventions such as information and support groups, and effective systems such as the overall care delivered through clinics. An important observation is that investigators demonstrated some degree of improvement in their subjects' health knowledge, attitude, or behavior.

Client Health Status

Patients who represented five major diagnostic classifications were subjects for an evaluation of a nurse clinic at the University of Kansas (Lewis & Resnick, 1967). The purpose of the clinic was to define the interprofessional roles of nursing and medicine in order to provide efficient care to large numbers of patients. For 1 year, 33 patients were randomly assigned to be cared for in the nurse clinic (experimental condition) and an additional 33 demographically and medically similar patients were randomly assigned to be cared for in the physician clinic (control condition). Compared with the physician clinic, patients in the nurse clinic: (a) reported a marked shift in their preference for nurses to perform certain procedures such as explain results ($X^2 = 9.09$, $p < 0.01$), explain tests ($X^2 = 12.5$, $p < 0.001$) and explain "what is wrong" ($X^2 = 12.07$, $p < 0.001$); (b) had fewer incidents of seeking medical attention for minor complaints; (c) reduced their frequency of complaints; (d) had a lower missed appointment rate (5% compared to a 10% in the physician clinic; (e) waited an average of 5.5 minutes compared with 58 minutes in the physician clinic; (f) had fewer hospital days than those in the physician clinic (34.2 days/1000 patients compared to 126.1 days/1000 patients); and (g) had lower costs ($2,475 for nurse clinic, versus $3,740 for physician group) and shorter lengths of stay when they were hospitalized (45 days for nurse group versus 68 days for physician group).

Lewis and Resnick (1967) used data collection and analysis procedures such as chart reviews, patient interviews, and time and motion studies. The authors concluded that nurses can provide primary care that patients wanted and needed at their particular phase of illness. Further, the authors stated that the nurse was not assisting the physician but was providing primary care consistent with patient needs that focused on the person and family rather than the disease.

Allison (1973) based her research and practice on Orem's Self-Care theory. Using pretest and posttest survey methods, Allison reported that patients and health care staff at the Johns Hopkins Hospital Diabetic Management Nurse Clinic were satisfied with the quality of care. Additionally, using patients as their own controls ($N = 160$), she found that patients demonstrated increased control of blood sugar levels, improved healing of leg ulcers and infections, reduced hospital admissions, and a decreased no-show rate (from 35% to 9%). Lack of details presented in the study made it difficult to evaluate the conclusions.

Jones (1976) analyzed physical and psychosocial assessments of clients ($N = 167$) registered at the Nursing Center for Family Health Services in Long Island, New York and individuals ($N = 328$) from the Moxey Rigby Housing Project. She identified the major health deficiencies for each age group, using a developmental approach.

Based on a subsample of 14 elderly, she found the major health problems to be hypertension, poor dietary habits, diabetes, arthritis, depression, visual defects, circulatory and dental. Her sample of 100 middle-aged adults (mainly women aged 45 to 64) revealed the following health problems: hypertension, severe dental concerns, nutritional problems, visual defects, menopausal complaints, role identity crises, reproductive pathology, gastric distress, and complaints of headaches, backaches, and nervousness.

The 43 young adults presented the following problems: single-parent responsibilities, sexual problems, poor nutrition, dental problems, limited social outlets, psychosomatic complaints, borderline hypertension, emotional problems, and alcoholism. Adolescents (N = 125) were found to have: severe dental decay, acne and skin rashes, poor nutrition and personal hygiene, outdated immunizations, alcohol and drug use, visual defects, and antisocial behavior problems. Few physical problems were found among the infants and children; the infants and children presented with upper respiratory infections, gastric upsets, skin rashes, dental problems, and slow development.

For each group of problems in the study, Jones (1976) made multidisciplinary, community-based recommendations. A better description of the sample and the assessment techniques would have improved the generalizability of her findings. However, this study provided an important, early description of the types of clients, problems, and care modalities that existed in nursing centers. Further, it contributed to the knowledge on which nursing practice is based.

Using health status as an outcome, Newman, Sloss, and Anderson (1984) evaluated the Louisville Visiting Nurses Association's Preventive Health Program. The program included 20 clinics located in public and private residences on a walk-in basis for persons over 60 years old. Services included health history and assessment of body systems; primary, secondary, and tertiary health activities; and special health events such as pap smear and breast self-examination clinics, influenza prevention, and glaucoma, diabetes, and hypertension screening. Policy was made by the Visiting Nurses Association and its board. Seventy-five percent of the board were consumers. The program was supported by funds from the federal government, county department of public health, and the United Way.

Data were collected on the following variables: cost per client visit; demographic profiles of clinic users including age, gender, education, marital status, living arrangements, income, race; use profiles including most common medical condition, referral source, average length of visit, average number of visits per client, most common referral by clinic, most common reason for leaving the service; and client satisfaction.

The first goal of the program was that of early detection of disease and prompt referral. Newman et al. (1984) presented the number of clients screened in two consecutive years, the percentage found to have a positive screening test, and the percentage with a confirmed diagnosis after being referred. These data were compared with national or state comparison data to calculate expected positives. Examples of the national data reported included the National Health Screening Council for hypertension and glaucoma, the Disease Detection Information Bureau for diabetes, and the Kentucky Department for Human Resources for hemoccult and cervical cancer. The screening program's outcome data were judged to be in line with outcomes from similar screening programs.

The second goal of the program was the prevention of health problems and complications from existing chronic conditions. This goal was evaluated by comparing the number of annual physician visits by clients with the average number of physician visits by others in the community. Data were available on only 20% (N = 493) of the clients. An earlier study (Human Services Coordination Alliance, 1976) in the Louisville area revealed that noninstitutionalized older adults visited their physician an average of 4.4 times per year and 25% did not make a physician visit at all. The clinic sample was found to make an average of 3.3 visits annually with only 4% making no visit. Thus, they concluded that clients in their sample were seeing medical doctors regularly but not excessively.

Newman, Sloss, and Anderson (1984) made a significant contribution to the literature and knowledge base for nursing centers. The strength of the design was in defining the nursing center data set to make it comparable with national, state, and local data sets for comparisons.

Nichols (1985a) studied clients of the Yale Midwifery Service (N = 175) regarding demographic characteristics and prenatal, intrapartum, postpartum, and neonatal variables. She found that most of the clientele were married, insured, or self-paying middle class, and experiencing a planned pregnancy. Nichols reported that 76% of the clients were delivered by a midwife, over an intact perineum in 43% of the cases, and without analgesia in 80% of the cases. Ninety-seven percent of the neonates had an Apgar score greater than 7, the mean birthweight was 3374 g, and 98% were breastfed. There was a 5% cesarean rate. This research served as a data base for comparability among nurse midwifery services. In comparison to other midwifery services, (Mann, 1981; Olsen, 1979) these outcomes were judged as excellent. Nichols contributed to the profile of the nursing center client and the database for nurse midwifery.

Nichols (1985b) also developed and tested a protocol for the evaluation and treatment of postdate pregnancy at the Yale Nurse Midwifery practice. Nichols found a rate of 10% "postdates" on the same 75 clients. The incidence of postmaturity, however, was only 3%. Based on her analysis of 17 "postdates" cases, Nichols developed a protocol for the management and care of the pregnant woman and her fetus at risk for postmaturity. Nichols did not address the reliability, validity, or other methods of protocol testing. However, the development of treatment protocols based on the literature and clinical experience is an example of the potential for research and practice in a nursing center.

To identify the most frequently occurring nursing diagnoses, Fehring and Frenn (1986) conducted a chart audit at the Marquette University Wellness

Resource Center. The five most frequently occurring diagnoses were: health maintenance—blood pressure; alteration in nutrition—greater than body requirements; anxiety—moderate; stress related to unemployment; and ineffective stress management. These findings are congruent with Jones' (1976) developmental analyses. Based on their audit, Fehring and Frenn presented a protocol for the nursing care of clients with a nursing diagnosis of health maintenance: blood pressure.

Riesch (1988) assessed a sample of 100 expectant mothers and their coaches enrolled in classes at the University of Wisconsin-Milwaukee Nursing Center to detect changes in their exercise of self-care agency before and after childbirth preparation classes. The sample was representative of the Milwaukee community with respect to race, marital status, education, and employment status. Both mothers and coaches demonstrated a significant increase in their attitudes toward exercising self-care as measured by scores on the Exercise of Self Care Agency scale after the sessions. Cronbach's alpha for the Self Care Agency scale was 0.865 for the study. Based on these data, Riesch recommended that childbirth preparation be included as part of a comprehensive prenatal health care package. A limitation of this study was the lack of a control group.

Jamieson and Martinson (1988) developed the Block Nurse program in St. Paul, Minnesota to serve the elderly who wanted to stay in their own homes and avoid "inappropriate hospitalization or nursing home placement." Using a system of nurses who resided in neighborhoods, home health and homemaking services were provided and closely monitored. After 4 years, Jamieson and Martinson reported that 85% of the Block Nurse clients would have been hospitalized without the program, the cost of providing the Block Nurse program was 24% less than the minimum cost of a nursing home, and family involvement in the care of the elderly relative was increased for clients in the Block Nurse program.

Each of the studies that included health status as a variable had methodological flaws, such as small samples, obscure instrumentation with poor reporting of psychometric properties, and lack of comparison groups. However, results suggest that nursing center care is cost effective, that investigators are attempting to measure effects of the care on patient outcomes and cost of care, and that care can be compared in terms of outcome to previously developed data bases.

Client Satisfaction

Nearly every report of research on nursing centers included some aspect of client satisfaction. The studies reviewed here are those limited to client satisfaction.

Using survey methods, Hill (1986) evaluated clients' satisfaction with care at the Leeds General Infirmary rheumatology clinic. She found that the clients perceived they were getting more individual and personal attention in the nurse clinic than they did in their previous experiences. Additionally, the subjects ($N = 35$) stated they benefitted from the nurses' referrals and explanations of arthritis aids and appliances. They responded that the nurses' teaching about the disease, its progression and side effects, and pain management was very helpful. Hill recommended that direct access to this type of nursing care be available to all patients rather than only to those enrolled in specialty clinics.

Client satisfaction was defined by Gresham-Kenton and Wisby (1987) to include clients': (a) perceptions that staff suggestions for health improvement were helpful, (b) recommendation of the service to others, (c) plans to continue to use the service, and (d) analysis of the number of hours the facility was available, comprehensiveness of the facility services, and comfort of the facility. Based on the instrument they developed and published for use by others, Gresham-Kenton and Wisby found their clients to be highly satisfied. They used the findings to change the clinic services; the clients' recommended more space and more extensive laboratory testing.

Based on an analysis of prior client satisfaction studies, Riesch (1985) suggested a structure, process, and outcome framework for the analysis of client satisfaction. Structure included comfort, accessibility, and convenience of the clinic rooms, location, hours, and fees. Process included the activities of the clinic such as assessment, support groups, classes, or screening clinics. Outcome included knowledge, attitude, or behavior changes made or intended, and objective health outcomes such as days lost from work or school, visits to physicians, emergency rooms, or hospitalizations.

Bagwell (1987) published the results of her survey of client satisfaction conducted at the Clemson University Nursing Center. She developed the instrument based on the literature and her clinical experience, had it reviewed by a panel of experts, and used it in a pilot study. No data regarding psychometric properties were reported. Based on her preliminary study, she developed two versions, one targeted for adults and one targeted for children under 16 years of age. The scale had 16 items concerning issues of courtesy by staff, respect for privacy, staff competence, satisfaction with amount of time and attention by staff, level of personal goal achievement, waiting time, and whether the client recommended the center to others. She documented a high level of satisfaction among her clients and identified areas for improvement for staff among the parents in her sample.

These studies have served to document what areas should be included in an assessment of client satisfaction. Based on these studies, it can be concluded that clients generally are satisfied with nursing center care.

Cost Effectiveness and Quality of Care

Kos and Rothberg (1981) were the only researchers who attempted to measure cost-effectiveness, utilization outcomes, and quality of care. By their own admission, the cost effectiveness analysis was somewhat simplistic, based on number of working days per year, number of clinic visits per year, and direct operating expenditures. They found an average cost of $42 per visit, compared with public health nurse costs, HMO costs, emergency room costs, and other published costs ranging from $37.50 to $50 per visit. Kos and Rothberg stated that the 1.8 staff usually saw an average of 5.5 patients per day. They felt this was less than full utilization and attributed this to poor transportation, geographic isolation, and a small patient pool.

To determine the quality of care, Kos and Rothberg described how the Nursing Center for Family Health Services instituted a formal evaluation by the Department of Community Health of the Albert Einstein College of Medicine [Morehead et al. (study) cited in Kos & Rothberg, 1981]. The evaluation included site visits by two physicians, two nurses, and a social worker. The Einstein team reportedly used standardized assessments of organizational structure and medical care systems. Kos and Rothberg did not define and describe the measures or assessments in the report. The team found that the Center was above average on preventive care ratings, exceedingly high on pediatric scores, and slightly below average on medicine and obstetrics. The team concluded that when compared with more traditional, physician-dominated organizations, the service "was not found wanting" (p. 32).

The Nursing Center for Health and Family Services closed despite the delivery of high quality health care as evidenced by the clients and the external audit team. Kos and Rothberg (1981, p. 35) stated the "reimbursement system was nonresponsive . . . attempts to interface with other provider systems were often thwarted, and we were unable to produce a large enough patient or client pool to generate sufficient income to cover costs." The authors concluded their research by quoting Guttentag's (1973, p. 39) assertion that to change health policy and systems one must "Use money for leverage, not services."

CONCLUSIONS AND RECOMMENDATIONS

This review of studies on nursing centers revealed that most centers have the goals of serving as a site for faculty and student research and basing practice on research, yet few studies have been conducted in or about nursing centers. The studies conducted had the following characteristics: (a) most studies lacked a theoretical or conceptual framework; (b) a variety of methods, that is, survey, quasi-experimental, case study, were used; (c) samples were small and mainly those of convenience or judgment, though representativeness of the community from which they were drawn was obtained in some studies; (d) the samples were varied but composed mainly of female, low income, healthy health care seekers; (e) research variables and their measurement were poorly defined; (f) control conditions were lacking in most instances, though data were comparable to other studies if carefully collected and analyzed; (g) data generally were gathered from only one center at a time using one method at a time; (h) there was no analysis of long-term or lag effects; (i) most of the methods were quantitative, representing little of the nursing center clients' lived experiences; and (j) there were no reports of replication of any previous studies. Thus, there is extensive untapped potential for research in nursing centers.

Barger (1987) viewed the nursing center as an entity to bridge the gap between research and practice. She identified the following components as conducive to research: (a) control of the practice; (b) economics of time and effort to integrate the practice and research roles, using the Duffy and Halloran (1987) study as an example; (c) computerization of nursing center databases; and (d) the academic environment, in which many of the centers reside, as a climate of innovation with a constant flow of fresh ideas.

To increase knowledge generation and use of nursing centers, multisite, multimethod, and clinical trials studies should be proposed, funded, and conducted. For example, many centers have protocols for patient care that should be analyzed for scientific adequacy. National and international studies should be conducted to: (a) develop and test computerized databases for client characteristics, nursing process, and outcomes that would serve the informational needs of the centers; (b) identify the outcomes nursing centers were developed to achieve; and (c) analyze the centers' cost effectiveness, efficiency, and quality of care.

To the extent that they are positive in comparison with outcomes of other health care providers, the outcomes of care in nursing centers could be used to support the case for reimbursement for nursing care and to develop health policy. Further, continuous study of the location and purposes of nursing centers should be accomplished, possibly by the National League for Nursing's Council on Nursing Centers. It would be useful to replicate Barger's demographic profile of nursing centers every 5 to 7 years in order to monitor the issues of location, purpose, and faculty practice.

Although the cross settings and multisite, multimethod, clinical trial studies will serve to document the larger issues of the scientific bases for care and subsequent outcomes, cost-effectiveness, efficiency, and quality, the value of the single case study, the clinical evaluation, and student research should not be forgotten. These centers serve as excellent sites for pilot studies, intervention studies, and numerous studies to document the experiences of care recipients.

REFERENCES

Allison, S. E. (1973). A framework for nursing action in a nurse-conducted diabetic management clinic. *Journal of Nursing Administration, 3*(4), 53–60.

Arlton, D. M., & Miercort, O. S. (1980). A nursing clinic: The challenge for student learning opportunities. *Journal of Nursing Education, 19*(1), 53–58.

Bagwell, M. A. (1987). Client satisfaction with nursing center services. *Journal of Community Health Nursing, 4,* 29–42.

Baird, S. C., & Benner, R. (1985). Keeping a university well with a health promotion clinic. *Nursing and Health Care, 6,* 107–109.

Barger, S. E. (1986a). Academic nurse-managed centers: Issues of implementation. *Family and Community Health, 9*(1), 12–22.

Barger, S. E. (1986b). Academic nursing centers: A demographic profile. *Journal of Professional Nursing, 2,* 246–251.

Barger, S. E. (1987). The potential for resources and research use in academic nurse-managed center. *Nurse Educator, 12*(6), 19–22.

Brown, N., Muhlenkamp, A., Fox, L., & Osborn, M. (1983). The relationship among health beliefs, health values, and health promotion activities. *Western Journal of Nursing Research, 5,* 155–163.

Burgess, W. (1988). *The resurgence of nursing centers: 1967–1987.* Milwaukee: University of Wisconsin-Milwaukee, Nursing Center.

Chickadonz, G. H., Burke, M. M., Fitzgerald, S., & Osterweis, M. (1982). Development of a primary care setting for nursing education. *Nursing and Health Care, 3,* 83–87, 92.

Dock, L. L. (1983c/1949). Relation of training schools to hospitals. In L. A. Hampton (Ed.), *Nursing of the Sick: 1893* (Reissued ed., pp 12–24). New York: McGraw Hill.

Duffy, D., & Halloran, M. C. (1987). Effect of an educational program on parents of children with asthma. *Childrens' Health Care, 16,* 76–81.

Fehring, R. J., & Frenn, M. (1986). Nursing diagnosis in a nurse-managed wellness resource center. In M. E. Hurley (Ed.), *Classification of nursing diagnoses: Proceedings of the Sixth Conference* (pp. 401–407). St. Louis, MO.: Mosby.

Fehring, R. J., Schulte, J., & Riesch, S. K. (1987). Toward a definition of nurse-managed centers. *Journal of Community Health Nursing, 3,* 59–67.

Glass, L. K. (1988, May). *The historic origins of nursing centers.* Paper presented at the meeting of the Fourth Biennial Conference on Nursing Centers, Milwaukee, WI.

Gresham-Kenton, X., & Wisby, M. (1987). Development and implementation of nurse-managed health program: A problem-oriented approach. *Journal of Ambulatory Care Management, 10,* 20–29.

Guttentag, M. (1973). Subjectivity and its use in program evaluation. *Evaluation, 1,* 60–65.

Hall, L. E. (1963). A center for nursing. *Nursing Outlook, 11,* 805–806.

Hauf, B. J. (1977). An evaluative study of a nursing center for community health nursing student experiences. *Journal of Nursing Education, 16*(8), 7–11.

Hawkins, J. W., Igou, J. F., Johnson, E. E., & Utley, Q. E. (1984). A nursing center for ambulatory, well, older adults. *Nursing and Health Care, 5,* 209–212.

Henry, O. M. (1978, October). *Demonstration centers for nursing practice, education, and research.* Paper presented at the meeting of the American Public Health Association, Los Angeles.

Higgs, Z. R. (1985). Carry the water to the desert. *Journal of Professional Nursing, 1,* 217–220.

Hill, J. (1986). Patient evaluation of a rheumatology nursing clinic. *Nursing Times, 82,* 42–43.

Human Services Coordination Alliance (1976). *Let older people speak for themselves: An assessment of need in KIDPA area developmental district.* Louisville, KY: The Alliance.

Jamieson, M., & Martinson, I. (1988, May). *The Block Nurse Program: Neighbors helping neighbors.* Paper presented at the meeting of the Fourth Biennial Conference on Nursing Centers, Milwaukee, WI.

Jones, A. (1976). Overview of a nursing center for family health services in Freeport. *Nurse Practitioner, 1*(1), 26–31.

Kaplan, C., & Cowles, A. (1978). Health locus of control and health values in the prediction of smoking reduction. *Health Education Monographs, 6,* 129–137.

Kinlein, M. L. (1972). Independent nurse practitioner. *Nursing Outlook, 20,* 22–24.

Kogan, H. N., Beaton, R., Betrus, P., Burr, R., Larson, M. L., Mitchell, P., & Wolf-Wilets, V. (1983). Nursing in transition: New structures, new practices, and new consumer responses. *Washington State Journal of Nursing, 54*(2), 37–41.

Kos, B. A., & Rothberg, J. S. (1981). Evaluation of a freestanding nurse clinic. In L. H. Aiken (Ed.), *Health policy and nursing practice* (pp. 19–42). New York: McGraw Hill.

Lenehan, G. P., McInnis, B. N., O'Donnell, D., & Hennessey, M. (1985). A nurses' clinic for the homeless. *American Journal of Nursing, 85,* 1237–1240.

Lewis, C. E., & Resnick, B. A. (1967). Nurse clinics and progressive ambulatory patient care. *New England Journal of Medicine, 277,* 1236–1241.

Lundeen, S. P. (1985). An interdisciplinary nurse-managed center: The Erie Family Health Center. In M. D. Mezey & D. O. McGivern (Eds.), *Nurses, Nurse Practitioners* (pp. 278–288). Boston: Little, Brown.

Mann, R. (1981). San Francisco General Hospital nurse midwifery practice: The first thousand births. *American Journal of Obstetrics and Gynecology, 140,* 167.

Mezey, M., & Chiamulera, D. N. (1980). Implementation of a campus nursing and health center in the baccalaureate curriculum. Part I: Overview of the center. *Journal of Nursing Education, 19*(5), 7–10.

Milio, N. (1970). *9226 Kercheval.* Ann Arbor, MI. University of Michigan Press.

Muhlenkamp, A. F., Brown, N. J., & Sands, D. (1985). Determinants of health promotion activities in nursing clinic clients. *Nursing Research, 34,* 327–332.

Munroe, D., & Natale, P. (1982). After-hours call in a primary care nursing practice. *Nurse Practitioner, 7*(5), 24–27.

Newman, J., Sloss, G. S., & Anderson, S. (1984). Evaluation of a health program. *Geriatric Nursing, 5,* 234–238.

Nichols, C. W. (1985a). The Yale Nurse Midwifery practice: Addressing the outcomes. *Journal of Nurse-Midwifery, 30,* 159–165.

Nichols, C. W. (1985b). Postdate pregnancy: Part II clinical implications. *Journal of Nurse-Midwifery, 30,* 259–268.

Olsen, L. (1979). Portrait of nurse-midwifery patients in a private practice. *Journal of Nurse-Midwifery, 24*(4), 10–17.

Ossler, C. C., Goodwin, M. E., Mariani, M., & Gilliss, C. L. (1982). Establishment of a nursing clinic for faculty and student clinical practice. *Nursing Outlook, 30,* 402–405.

Resolutions. (1925). *The Kentucky Committee for Mothers and Babies Quarterly Bulletin, 1*(2), 15–16.

Riesch, S. K. (1985). A primary care initiative: Nurse-managed centers. In M. D. Mezey & D. O. McGivern (Eds.), *Nurses, Nurse Practitioners* (pp. 242–248). Boston: Little, Brown.

Riesch, S. K. (1988). Changes in the exercise of self-care agency: Childbearing dyad. *Western Journal of Nursing Research, 10,* 257–266.

Riesch, S. K., Fehring, R. J., Schulte, J. A., & Wright, N. A. (1986, April). *State of the art of research in nurse-managed centers.* Paper presented at the meeting of the Third Biennial Conference on Nursing Centers, Scottsdale, AZ.

Riesch, S., Felder, E., & Stauder, C. (1980). Nursing centers can promote health for individuals, families, and communities. *Nursing Administration Quarterly, 4*(3), 1–8.

Sanger, M. (1971). *Margaret Sanger: An autobiography.* New York: Dover (reprint of 1938 by W. W. Norton).

Thibodeau, J. A., & Hawkins, J. (1987). Evolution of a nursing center. *Journal of Ambulatory Care Management, 10,* 30–39.

Wallston, B. S., & Wallston, K. A. (1981). Health locus of control scales. In H. M. Lefcourt (Ed.). *Research with the locus of control construct. Vol. I: Assessment Methods* (pp. 189–243). New York: Academic Press.

Woolf, S. J. (1937, March 7). Miss Wald at 70 sees her dreams realized. *New York Times Magazine.*

PART III

Research on Nursing Education

Chapter 9

Nursing Administration Education

RUTH A. ANDERSON
SCHOOL OF NURSING
UNIVERSITY OF TEXAS AT AUSTIN

CONTENTS

One hundred years ago Miss E. P. Davis, Superintendent of the University of Pennsylvania Hospital, suggested that nurses moving into management roles should possess a specialized body of knowledge to complement their nursing expertise (Davis, 1893). It was not until the 1950s, though, that nursing administration education programs began to proliferate in the United States (Mullane, 1959). In that decade there were farsighted attempts to define the educational requirements of nurse administrators and suggestions that administrative science be taught as a core component of nursing administration educational programs (Finer, 1952; Hamilton, 1949; Mullane, 1959). In the

1960s and early 1970s, however, graduate education in nursing emphasized clinical specialization and ignored education in nursing administration (Blair, 1976).

Beginning about 1974, concurrent with the rapid changes in health care technology and financing, there were renewed and enthusiastic efforts to develop graduate nursing administration programs. The number of programs tripled from 24 in 1974 to 74 in 1989 (Mark, Turner, & Englebardt, 1990). Throughout this period of rejuvenation, nurse educators have suggested that nursing administration education be interdisciplinary in nature, including both business administration (Blair, 1989; Fine, 1978; Henry, 1989a; Mark et al., 1990; McCloskey, Gardner, Johnson, & Maas, 1988; McClure, 1985; Poulin, 1979; Price, 1984; Simms, 1988; Stevens, 1978) and public administration (Henry, 1989b).

This review and critique of research includes studies related to nursing administration education from 1970 through 1989. Studies were reviewed if they contained empirical findings that addressed (a) curriculum, including studies of skills essential to the effective practice of nursing administration; (b) program effectiveness; (c) nursing administration education as part of clinical education programs; and (d) doctoral education in nursing administration.

Computer database searches of MEDLINE from 1983 to 1989 and of Health Administration and Planning from 1975 to 1989 were done under a variety of subject headings such as nursing administration education, nursing education research, nursing education, graduate nursing education, curriculum, nurse administrators, and administrative personnel. Because the computer search yielded only eight relevant studies, a systematic search of selected nursing and related journal indexes was carried out manually. The annual indexes of *Journal of Nursing Administration; Journal of Nursing Education; Journal of Professional Nursing; Image: Journal of Nursing Scholarship; International Journal of Nursing Studies; Nurse Educator; Nursing Administration Quarterly; Nursing and Health Care; Nursing Economics; Nursing Management; Nursing Outlook; Nursing Research; Research in Nursing and Health;* and *Western Journal of Nursing Research* were searched from 1970 through 1989. Journals that did not date back to 1970 were searched from their inception. The manual search yielded 13 relevant articles in addition to the eight found by computer search. Nine articles appeared in *Journal of Nursing Administration;* four in *Journal of Nursing Education;* four in *Nursing Outlook;* two in *Nursing Administration Quarterly;* and one each in *Image: Journal of Nursing Scholarship* and *Nursing Economics*. Three articles were published before 1975, five between 1980 and 1985, and 13 between 1986 and 1989. The annual indexes of related journals, including *Health Care Management Review, Health Services Research, Hospital and*

Health Services Administration, Journal of Health Administration Education, and *Journal of Health and Human Resources Administration,* were searched back through 1970 but yielded no relevant articles.

In this integrative review, each article was abstracted using a procedure described by Schultz and Miller (1990). Substantive content for each article was organized according to purpose, framework, design, sample, instrumentation, procedures, data analysis, results, and implications. A judgment about replicability was formed by the reviewer on the basis of the study's quality and detail as inferred from the report. To facilitate analysis, the data from the articles were entered into a text database using the computer program *MaxThink* (Larson, 1990).

The 21 articles were grouped into four categories: curricular content; program structure, characteristics, and effectiveness; nursing administration education as part of clinical education programs; and doctoral education. Three studies (Price, 1984; Reynolds, 1987; Wagner, Henry, Giovinco, & Blanks, 1988) addressed both curricular content and program effectiveness, but for the purposes of this review the articles are discussed in the section that best reflects the primary purpose of the research. A synthesis of research findings is reported for the studies in each category, followed by an integrative critique of the research.

Although the number of studies on nursing administration education has increased over the last 15 years, the recent proliferation in the number of nursing administration programs would lead one to expect an even larger body of empirical research. It is possible that the number of studies is low because only relatively recently has the acceptance of nursing administration as a legitimate area for graduate study in nursing emerged. It also may be due to a lack of funding sources for educational research and to the substantial shortage of faculty for teaching and research in this area (Henry, 1989c). Research on education in nursing administration may be conducted more frequently than the literature reflects but may not be published because of a lack of outlets. This position is suggested by the observation that 5 of the 21 articles in this review (Damewood, 1988; Marriner-Tomey, 1989a, 1989b; Stepura & Tilbury, 1988; Vance & Wolf, 1986) appeared as abstracts or briefs.

CURRICULAR CONTENT

Ten studies were focused on the knowledge and skills needed to be an effective nurse administrator (NA), suggesting curricular content needs. The studies are discussed under three categories: clinical nursing, nursing administration, and general administration. Studies are discussed under the heading of clinical nursing if they included concepts for study related to general or specialized clinical knowledge in nursing. Studies are discussed under the heading nursing administration if the findings included concepts for study that require specific knowledge of nursing and health care, even though they may build on a foundation of knowledge in general administration. Studies are discussed under the heading of general administration when the findings comprised concepts for study that require administrative knowledge not specific to nursing and health care.

Clinical Nursing

Whether expert clinical nursing knowledge and skill are required by NAs long has been debated. Two studies reported that NAs in long-term care settings use clinical knowledge and skill more than NAs in other settings. As part of a larger 3-year study of 40 nursing homes in the Detroit area, Barney (1974) used observation and interview techniques to study NA roles. The NAs frequently were called upon for their clinical nursing expertise as they were often the "only full-time professional with authority" (Barney, 1974, p. 438). Simms, Price, and Pfoutz (1985) reported a study of 30 NAs in 10 acute-care institutions, 10 home-care agencies, and 10 long-term care facilities. Using a grounded-theory approach, they examined the role of the NA in each setting. In nursing homes, NAs had a major responsibility for direct care, often covering when short of staff, participating in patient care conferences, working with families, and providing clinical consultation.

In four studies researchers addressed the question of whether clinical expertise is needed by NAs in hospital or home health care settings. Freund (1985) conducted a study of 172 NAs and 126 chief executive officers (CEOs) in randomly selected university-affiliated hospitals to identify what makes an effective nurse administrator. Moore, Biordi, Holm, and McElmurry (1988), using a randomly selected sample of 289 NAs and 166 CEOs from community hospitals, replicated Freund's (1985) study. Poulin (1984) conducted interviews with 12 NAs, selected because they had been identified by peers as being competent and progressive in their roles. She examined the role functions and competencies required for effectiveness. Freund (1985), Moore et al. (1988), Poulin (1984), and Simms et al. (1985) found in acute-care settings that clinical expertise was not stressed as a skill necessary for effectiveness of NAs in their roles; findings similar to those found by Simms et al. (1985) in home care settings.

Nursing Administration Content

Respondents in four studies indicated that knowledge and skill are needed for creating and maintaining nursing systems of care, including setting and implementing standards of care (Poulin, 1984; Simms et al., 1985), ensuring control mechanisms (Poulin, 1984), maintaining patient care quality (Simms et al., 1985), providing necessary human and material resources (Poulin, 1984), developing and disseminating personnel policies (Poulin, 1984), and developing staffing plans (Barney, 1974; Poulin, 1984; Simms et al., 1985).

Wagner et al. (1988) did a content analysis of 37 articles in *Journal of Nursing Administration, Nursing Administration Quarterly,* and *Nursing Outlook* that met their titling criteria. They also analyzed all the works of Blair, Poulin, and Stevens for the purpose of identifying published suggestions for nursing administration education. Titling criteria included the following terms or some variation of these terms: "director of nursing, nurse manager, nurse executives, or nurse administrators, combined with the terms education, preparation, or implications for education" (p. 211). Wagner et al. (1988) found published suggestions to comprise nursing theory, environments, health-care-delivery settings, systems designs, health-care technology, and community, societal, and consumer health needs.

In five studies, researchers identified a need for a general knowledge of: (a) patient-care services such as home-care clinics and alcoholic rehabilitation (Poulin, 1984), (b) departments other than nursing (Simms et al., 1985), (c) developing and maintaining medical staff relationships (Freund, 1985; Moore et al., 1988), and (d) community health needs (Poulin, 1984; Wagner et al., 1988). In two studies researchers found that NAs have an extensive role in education. Pfoutz, Simms, and Price (1987) examined the data obtained in the study reported by Simms et al. (1985) to gain an understanding of the NA's role in education. Nurse administrators in all settings reported having a major role in education. This role involved mentor relationships, staff development, program development, educational services, and, to a lesser extent, direct teaching. The nurse administrators also reported playing a major educational role outside their own organizations through lectures and presentations. The NAs reported an increasing need for proposal-writing skills. Poulin (1984) also reported that NAs had a major responsibility for education, including educating their departmental staffs, serving as preceptors, teaching classes in schools of nursing, and guest lecturing. The findings of these two studies suggest that programs should include content on public speaking, proposal writing, program development and evaluation, and teaching and learning theory.

Knowledge and skill in research were identified as necessary for NAs by respondents in four studies. In a study of 40 NAs and educators selected as an advisory panel to identify the topics most important for study by nurse managers, Vance and Wolf (1986) identified evaluation methods as one of 15 areas of knowledge essential for NAs. Research was mentioned in 26 of 37 publications as suggested content for study (Wagner et al., 1988). Research frequently is offered in nursing administration programs, as Stepura and Tilbury (1988) found in their analysis of the curriculum of 64 programs in nursing administration at 54 schools. In the Simms et al. (1985) study, NAs viewed their role as one of facilitating research rather than one of direct participation.

In two studies researchers examined the state of the art in nursing administration education using content analysis techniques. In an analysis of curriculum in 64 programs in nursing administration, Stepura and Tilbury (1988) found that generic course content consisted of nursing theory, theory development, professional issues, leadership, health care systems, and role theory. Marriner-Tomey (1989a) content analyzed 23 nursing administration textbooks to identify the theories being used to teach nursing administration and found that needs and goals theories of motivation and theories of leadership were the most extensively covered topics. She also concluded that many of the books were atheoretical.

General Administration Content

Respondents in six studies identified general knowledge of finance, accounting, and economics as necessary. Wagner et al. (1988) reported suggestions for content in finance, including economics, costing, and reimbursement, in over 50% of the articles reviewed. Freund (1985) found that knowledge of general management, health, and nursing was the most frequently cited reason for the NA effectiveness by CEOs and NAs at university-affiliated hospitals. General management knowledge, which included knowing about finance, accounting, and computer operations, was believed to be as important as knowledge of health and nursing. Moore et al. (1988), in a replication of Freund's study, found that knowledge of general management, health, and nursing was ranked third as a reason for the NA effectiveness by CEOs and NAs at community hospitals. Poulin (1984) and Simms et al. (1985) found that NAs reported controlling large budgets and large staffs. Nurse administrators in acute care and home care settings, however, participated more frequently in budget development than did NAs in long-term care (Simms et al., 1985). The Vance and Wolf (1986) advisory panel of NAs and educators ranked fiscal management as the most important of 15 topics for study by nurse managers.

Skill in human management and knowledge of organizational behavior and theory were identified in eight studies as essential for NAs. Human-management skill was ranked as the most important characteristic of effective NAs by respondents in the Moore et al. (1988) study; it was the second most frequently cited reason for effectiveness in Freund's (1985) study. An NA's flexibility and ability to negotiate and compromise were ranked fifth by the respondents in the Moore et al. (1988) study, and sixth in Freund's (1985) study as reasons for NA effectiveness. In acute care settings, Simms et al.

(1985) found that union-related and collective-bargaining activities were major responsibilities. Simms et al. (1985) found that leadership behaviors were reported to be important for effectivenss in all settings. In the Vance and Wolf (1986) study, 12 of the 15 topics identified as most important for study by nurse managers related to human management skill, organizational behavior, and organizational theory. The need for political savvy was reported to be essential by 22.1% of the university-affiliated hospital NAs in Freund's (1985) study, while only 4% of CEOs reported this to be essential for effectiveness. Political savvy was seen as important by only 2% of NAs and 1% of CEOs in community hospitals (Moore et al., 1988). Wagner et al. (1988) found suggestions for content in organizational theory; organizational behavior; decision making and problem solving; leadership and power; motivation; group process; accountability, conflict, cooperation, and negotiation; and planning, directing, or coordinating. Stepura and Tilbury (1988) found that 30 out of 66 programs in nursing administration required students to study administrative and organizational theories.

In three studies, researchers found that NAs have a role in the strategic management of health care organizations. Simms et al. (1985) reported that NAs in acute-care and home-care settings indicated that they had substantial roles in long-range planning and policy making. Possession of a total organizational view, necessary for strategic decision making, was cited third most frequently by CEOs and fourth most frequently by NAs as a reason for NA effectiveness in university-affiliated hospitals (Freund, 1985) and was ranked second by CEOs and fourth by NAs in community hospitals (Moore et al., 1988).

Computer knowledge was an area that the studies reviewed did not address to a great extent. Wagner et al. (1988) found that knowledge of management-information systems was suggested with increasing frequency from 1981 to 1985 as content for study in nursing administration. Freund (1985) found that computer literacy was mentioned by many CEOs and NAs as essential for effective NAs.

Integrative Critique

An examination of this research on curricular content indicates that a generally credible foundation for planning nursing administration educational programs is available. The research was descriptive in design, including descriptive survey (Freund, 1985; Moore et al. 1988; Stepura & Tilbury, 1988); descriptive exploratory (Barney, 1974; Poulin, 1984; Vance & Wolf, 1986); grounded theory (Pfoutz et al., 1987; Simms et al., 1985); and content analysis of the literature (Marriner-Tomey, 1989a; Wagner et al., 1988). Conceptual frameworks were identified in 6 of the 10 studies (Moore et al.,

1988; Pfoutz et al., 1987; Poulin, 1984; Simms et al., 1985; Vance & Wolfe, 1986; Wagner et al., 1988), although most relied heavily on management theory rather than nursing theory.

Random-sampling procedures were used in two studies (Freund, 1985; Moore et al., 1988). Systematic nonprobability sampling procedures were used in three studies. Pfoutz et al. (1987) and Simms et al. (1985) used purposeful, convenience sampling to obtain local and national representativeness of various nursing care settings. Poulin (1984) used purposeful, convenience sampling to obtain subjects identified by their peers as competent nurse administrators. In two studies the researchers attempted to include the whole population of interest: all schools offering academic preparation in nursing administration (Stepura & Tilbury, 1988) or all publications meeting titling or authorship criteria (Wagner et al., 1988). A convenience sample was used by researchers in two studies (Marriner-Tomey, 1989a; Vance & Wolf, 1986). Barney (1974) did not provide details of the sampling procedure used. Three studies (Freund, 1985; Moore et al., 1988; Stepura & Tilbury, 1988) were national in scope.

Descriptive statistics only were reported in one study (Moore et al., 1988). Content analyses or some type of qualitative analysis, often combined with descriptive statistics, were reported in seven studies (Freund, 1985; Marriner-Tomey, 1989a; Pfoutz et al., 1987; Poulin, 1984; Simms et al., 1985; Steptura & Tilbury, 1988; Wagner et al., 1988). Data analysis procedures were not well documented in two research reports (Barney, 1974; Vance & Wolfe, 1986).

The primary weakness of these studies was that the discussion of instrumentation often was absent. In seven studies (Barney, 1974; Freund, 1985; Moore et al., 1988; Pfoutz et al., 1987; Stepura & Tilbury, 1988; Simms et al., 1985; Vance & Wolf, 1986), the reliability or validity of data-collection instruments or content-analysis procedures were not specifically discussed. Of the three studies reporting validity or reliability, face validity was reported in one study (Poulin, 1984) and validity of the classification was reported in one study (Marriner-Tomey, 1989a). Wagner et al. (1988) reported semantic validity, a form of validity whereby coding during content analysis was based on a typology of concepts with common meaning among the coders of data, and sampling validity, which addressed the representativeness of the data. Four researchers adapted existing instruments (Moore et al., 1988; Pfoutz et al., 1987; Poulin, 1984; Simms et al., 1985) and five developed instruments for use in their studies (Freund, 1985; Marriner-Tomey, 1989a; Stepura & Tilbury, 1988; Vance & Wolf, 1986; Wagner et al., 1988).

Two studies (Barney, 1974; Vance & Wolf, 1986) were judged inadequate for replication because sampling procedures, data-collection procedures, and data-analysis procedures were not well described. The remaining eight studies were judged adequate for replication on the basis of the report.

PROGRAM STRUCTURE, CHARACTERISTICS, AND EFFECTIVENESS

The six studies discussed in this section include research in which investigators compared different program structures, addressed practica as part of programs of study, and examined program characteristics that led to student satisfaction or selection of programs.

Structure and Effectiveness

In four studies researchers examined program structures within schools of nursing. Price (1984) studied 141 graduates from three types of nursing master's programs, those with a major in: (a) nursing administration with a clinical specialization, (b) nursing administration without a clinical specialization, or (c) clinical specialization with an administrative component. All graduates held positions in nursing administration. Price, comparing each program's effectiveness in contributing to NAs' role performance, found statistically significant differences in the graduates' perceived ability to perform management, personnel, and budget roles. Graduates from programs in nursing administration, with or without clinical minors, felt more capable than graduates from clinical nursing programs with a minor in nursing administration. Price asked the employers (92 participated) of these 141 graduates to rate the graduates' role performance; there were no statistically significant differences in ratings of performance of the graduates from the three types of programs.

Duffy and Gold (1980) compared two groups of NAs, 43 with master's degrees in nursing administration and 33 with master's degrees in business, health care, or public administration. All were employed by hospitals with more than 200 beds. NAs with non-nursing administration degrees had significantly higher perceived preparation scores for budgeting, marketing, and statistics. Nurse administrators with nursing administration degrees had significantly higher perceived preparation scores for research and program inservice education skills. There were no significant differences on scores for 18 (78%) of the 23 managerial skills. Additionally, Duffy and Gold reported that the majority of respondents (65% of those with nursing administration degrees and 78% of those with non-nursing administration degrees) rated their perceived preparation for all 23 managerial skills below 4.5 or the midpoint of the scale, indicating that both types of programs need to strengthen their curricula.

Reynolds (1987) studied a randomly selected sample of 123 NAs in hospitals with more than 200 beds to examine how adequately they were prepared for their roles. Reynolds reported that out of 62 managerial responsibilities, areas relating to fiscal management and legal matters were the areas in which NAs experienced the most difficulty. Graduates from master's programs in nursing administration felt less prepared in these areas than graduates with MBAs or doctorates. They felt more prepared, however, than did graduates from nonMBA, nonnursing administration programs. Reynolds does not report whether these differences were significant.

Scalzi and Anderson (1989a) surveyed a randomly selected sample of 103 NAs and 60 CEOs to determine what they believed to be the best educational preparation for NAs. The majority, 75% of NAs and 65% of CEOs, chose the dual degree Masters of Science in Nursing (MSN)/Masters in Business Administration (MBA) as the best preparation for nursing administrators. The second most favored degree was the MSN with a business minor (17% of NAs and 33% of CEOs), followed by the PhD in nursing administration (8% of NAs and 2% of CEOs). When asked what degree would most improve their own marketability, 69% of NAs chose the MSN/MBA, 17% chose the MSN with a business minor, and 13% chose the PhD.

Practica

Practica or residencies were addressed in three studies. Practica and residencies have similar objectives, but residencies usually require a greater time commitment by students, who may also be paid. Damewood (1988) interviewed 11 clinical directors about their own educational experiences. She found that the respondents believed that the practicum was the most valuable requirement in their management curriculum and that it was best when the practicum accommodated individual career goals. Scalzi and Anderson (1989a) reported that the NAs ranked a paid administrative residency as the least important factor to consider when choosing a program. CEOs ranked the administrative residency last among important characteristics for evaluating nurse executive applicants. Stepura and Tilbury (1988) found that more than half of all 66 programs reviewed had administrative practicum experiences as part of the curriculum.

Program Characteristics

Researchers in three studies examined characteristics that students valued when selecting programs. Thomas, Erickson, and Heick (1974), in a study of

59 graduates of one program, found that factors cited as important in selection of the program were accreditation, stature of the university, and bulletin/catalog information (50%); location and availability of family and friends in the area (40%); and qualification of faculty (10%). Price (1984) found that 35% of 141 responding NAs were satisfied with their graduate programs, citing as reasons: curriculum design, expertise of faculty, and interdisciplinary approach. The reason cited for dissatisfaction was failure of the programs to prepare them adequately for administrative roles. Scalzi and Anderson (1989a) asked NAs to rank five factors in order of importance to them in the choice of a graduate program and found that reputation and location ranked closely as first and second in importance, whereas length of program and cost of tuition ranked closely as third and fourth.

Integrative Critique

Descriptive survey designs were used in two studies (Scalzi & Anderson, 1989a; Thomas et al., 1974), descriptive exploratory in one study (Damewood, 1988), and comparative, nonexperimental designs in three studies (Duffy & Gold, 1980; Price, 1984; Reynolds, 1987). In only one study was a conceptual framework reported (Price, 1984). Random sampling procedures were used in two studies (Reynolds, 1987; Scalzi & Anderson, 1989a). Systematic nonprobability sampling procedures were used in two studies. Price (1984) used a purposeful, stratified technique to identify schools that were representative of national geographic areas and types of master's programs in nursing administration. Duffy and Gold (1980) used snowballing to identify subjects. In one study the researcher attempted to include the whole population of interest: all of the graduates of a degree program (Thomas et al., 1974). A convenience sample was used by researchers in one study (Damewood, 1988). Three studies (Duffy & Gold, 1980; Price, 1984; Scalzi & Anderson, 1989a) were national in scope.

The reliability and validity of data-collection instruments or content-analysis procedures were not discussed in four studies (Damewood, 1988; Reynolds, 1987; Scalzi & Anderson, 1989a; Thomas et al., 1974). Although few details were given, pretesting was mentioned in one report (Duffy & Gold, 1980) and content validity was mentioned in one report (Price, 1984). One researcher adapted an existing instrument (Price, 1984) and four developed instruments for use in their studies (Duffy & Gold, 1980; Reynolds, 1987; Scalzi & Anderson, 1989a; Thomas et al., 1974).

Parametric statistics were used for data analysis in two studies (Duffy & Gold, 1980; Price, 1984). The use of parametric statistics by Duffy and Gold (1980) and Price (1984) was appropriate. Three studies reported descriptive statistics only (Reynolds, 1987; Scalzi & Anderson, 1989a; Thomas et al.,

1974). In one research report, data-analysis procedures were not well documented (Damewood, 1988).

Two studies (Damewood, 1988; Reynolds, 1987) were judged inadequate for replication because sampling procedures, data-collection procedures, and data-analysis procedures were not well described. Both Damewood (1988) and Reynolds (1987) drew conclusions that went beyond the data presented in the reports. The remaining four studies were judged adequate for replication on the basis of the report.

NURSING ADMINISTRATION CONTENT FOR CLINICAL EDUCATION PROGRAMS

In three studies researchers addressed clinical master's programs and reported findings that identified a need to develop nursing-administration content for clinical programs. Donley, Jepson, and Perloff (1973), in a study of 44 respondents from a master's program in clinical nursing, found that almost 60% would have preferred a program that included a functional minor in teaching, nursing administration, or both, because their positions required knowledge in these areas. Brophy, Rankin, Butler, and Egenes (1989) interviewed 23 NAs in 23 hospitals with psychiatric units to determine the employment market for nurses with master's degrees in mental health nursing. Twenty of the respondents stated that nursing-management content should be part of the graduate curricula in mental health nursing. The 23 hospitals employed 47 nurses who had master's degrees in mental health nursing; half of these were employed in some type of management role. Hill (1989) asked a convenience sample of 13 NAs and 34 staff nurses to project future trends in health care and to state which knowledge and skills they considered both critical for survival and best learned in master's programs. The respondents predicted that an understanding of economics and computers would be essential and indicated that content in business and management as well as legal and ethical issues should be part of master's curricula in nursing.

A descriptive survey design was used by Donley et al. (1973) and Hill (1989) and a descriptive exploratory design was used by Brophy et al. (1989). Donley et al. (1973) described a conceptual framework that was based on industrial engineering rather than nursing. No conceptual framework was reported by Brophy et al. (1989) or Hill (1989). In one study the researchers attempted to include the whole population of interest: all of the graduates of a degree program (Donley et al., 1973). A convenience sample was used by Brophy et al. (1989) and Hill (1989). Hill (1989) reported content validity and Brophy et al. (1989) reported face validity. Donley et al. (1973) did not report reliability or validity. Hill (1989) adapted existing instruments, whereas

Brophy et al. (1989) and Donley et al. (1973) developed instruments for use in their studies. Donley et al. (1973) and Hill (1989) reported descriptive statistics only. Brophy et al. (1989) reported content analysis with descriptive statistics. All studies were judged adequate for replication based on the report.

DOCTORAL EDUCATION

In two studies researchers addressed doctoral education in nursing administration. Marriner-Tomey (1989b) surveyed 22 schools with doctoral programs in nursing administration to determine what research topics were being studied. She found that the number of faculty doing related research ranged from one to nine and the number of related dissertations ranged from 0 to 21. Specific topics of the research were not identified due to a lack of retrieval mechanisms. Wiley (1989) surveyed 27 deans or directors of doctoral programs in schools that offered the PhD in Nursing. When asked what topics were accepted as dissertations, 67% indicated that they accepted topics in nursing administration as an appropriate area of study.

Both Wiley (1989) and Marriner-Tomey (1989b) used a descriptive survey design. Conceptual frameworks were not specified. The researchers in both studies attempted to include the whole population of interest: all schools with doctoral programs in nursing administration (Marriner-Tomey, 1989b) and all schools with doctoral programs in nursing (Wiley, 1989). Both studies were national in scope. There was no discussion of instrumentation or reliability and validity of data-collection instruments. In both studies the researchers developed their own instruments. Only descriptive statistics were reported, which was appropriate for the type of studies done. The studies were judged adequate for replication on the basis of the report.

SUMMARY AND RESEARCH DIRECTIONS

This integrative review demonstrated that there is a core of knowledge and skill needed by NAs in all health care settings. However, in different practice settings different knowledge and skills are emphasized. A better understanding of how these differences affect nursing administration curricula requires additional research to examine differences in practice across settings. For example, what program options are needed for nurses who plan careers in long-term care? Future researchers might examine the specific benefits that clinical experience gives NAs and at what career point this experience should occur. For example, what benefits are gained if students in nursing administration programs have had clinical nursing experience before their program of study? Can nurses effectively gain required clinical experience after completing a master's degree in nursing administration?

More research is needed on computer literacy for NAs. Peterson and Gerdin-Jelger (1988), in a book on nursing informatics, have suggested what computer competencies are needed by NAs. Research is needed on effective teaching strategies as well as on the required depth of understanding of the theories and principles underlying computer applications.

We may infer from the studies included in this review that the knowledge needed by NAs is both disciplinary and interdisciplinary (Blair, 1989; Henry, 1989a; Jennings & Meleis, 1988), and thus may best be obtained from interdisciplinary programs. The empirical findings do not, however, provide clear direction regarding how or with whom such interdisciplinary programs should be developed. Although NAs and CEOs view the dual degree MSN/MBA as the best preparation for nurse administrators, there is no empirical evidence to show that NAs with dual degrees perform more effectively. Thus, schools of nursing should take care when forming alliances with schools of administration. Further research should compare the effectiveness of dual-degree programs and nursing programs with other types of formal interdisciplinary relationships with schools of business administration, public administration, or health care administration. Future studies should move beyond opinion surveys about perceived preparation and performance to well-specified educational, program, and performance outcomes.

Findings on the value of practicum experiences in nursing administration curricula were mixed. Because practica can be expensive to students and health care organizations alike, this is an important area for further study. Directions for future research should include questions such as: What concepts and skills are learned and what benefits are gained by students in practicum experiences? What are the most effective practicum arrangements—full time for a shorter period or part time over longer periods? What teaching strategies are most effective to assist students to integrate theory and practice?

A few researchers suggested that nursing administration content is needed by graduates of clinical nursing programs. More research is needed for a better understanding of the roles of graduates of clinical nursing master's programs and the type of administrative knowledge and skills that would enhance their role performances.

Few researchers have evaluated doctoral education in nursing administration. Knowledge of curriculum development, however, might be gained from studies that examine conceptual and theoretical linkages between doctoral and master's programs in nursing administration and the differences between practice behaviors of NAs with master's degrees and those with doctorates.

No research included in this review addressed the selection of students or student characteristics that predict success in graduate education and subsequent practice. There was also no research that asked what administrative nursing content is useful for undergraduate nursing curricula. Both of these are areas for future research.

This integrative critique points out two weaknesses of previous research that should be addressed in future studies. First, many studies either lacked a conceptual framework or relied heavily on management theories. Schultz and Miller (1990), in a review of nursing-administration research, reported similar findings. An explanation of these findings may be that until recently not much theoretical work in nursing administration had been published. Recent theoretical work by authors such as Anderson and Scalzi (1989), Blair (1989), Henry (1989a), Jennings and Meleis (1988), Gardner, Kelly, Johnson, McCloskey, and Maas (1991), Neidlinger and Miller (1990), Nyberg (1990), Ray (1989), Scalzi and Anderson (1989b), and Schultz (1987) may be helpful for developing future research from a nursing perspective. A second critical problem in this body of research is that reliability and validity of data-collection instruments and qualitative-analysis procedures often were not reported. Perhaps this problem has resulted in part from the fact that several researchers developed instruments for their studies without the guidance of a conceptual or theoretical framework. More attention should be paid in future research to assessing and reporting the reliability and validity of instruments.

Overall, the studies in this review, being generally descriptive in nature, provide a foundation of knowledge on which to build programs of master's education in nursing administration. More studies are needed to evaluate the impact of different educational models on the effectiveness of nurse administrators' practice.

REFERENCES

Anderson, R. A., & Scalzi, C. S. (1989). A theory development role for nurse administrators. *Journal of Nursing Administration, 19*(5), 23–29.

Barney, J. L. (1974). Nursing directors in nursing homes. *Nursing Outlook, 22,* 436–440.

Blair, E. M. (1976). NAQ forum: What is needed in leadership for nursing administration? *Nursing Administration Quarterly, 1,* 68–69.

Blair, E. M. (1989). Nursing and administration: A synthesis model. *Nursing Administration Quarterly, 13*(2), 1–11.

Brophy, E. B., Rankin, D., Butler, S., & Egenes, K. (1989). The master's prepared mental health nurse: An assessment of employer expectations. *Journal of Nursing Education, 28,* 156–160.

Damewood, D. M. (1988). Targeting student learning at the critical skills of the middle manager. *Journal of Nursing Administration, 18*(3), 6, 38.

Davis, E. P. (1893). Trained nurses as superintendents of hospitals. In I. A. Hampton (Ed.), *Nursing of the sick, 1893: Papers and discussions from the International Congress of Charities, Correction and Philanthropy, Chicago, 1893* (pp. 106–110). Published in 1949 under the sponsorship of the National League of Nursing Education, New York: McGraw-Hill.
Donley, R., Jepson, V., & Perloff, E. (1973). Graduate education for practice realities. *Nursing Outlook, 21,* 646–649.
Duffy, M. E., & Gold, N. E. (1980). Education for nursing administration: What investment yields highest returns? *Journal of Nursing Administration, 10*(9), 31–38.
Fine, R. B. (1978). The clinical component of administrative practice in nursing to nursing administration. In C. Slater (Ed.), *The education and roles of nursing service administrators* (pp. 15–20). Battle Creek, MI: W. K. Kellogg Foundation.
Finer, H. (1952). *Administration and the nursing services.* New York: Macmillan.
Freund, C. M. (1985). Director of nursing effectiveness: DON and CEO perspective and implications for education. *Journal of Nursing Administration, 15*(6), 25–30.
Gardner, D., Kelly, K., Johnson, M., McCloskey, J. C., & Maas, M. (1991). Nursing administration model for administrative practice. *Journal of Nursing Administration, 21*(3), 37–41.
Hamilton, J. A. (1949). Success or failure in nursing administration? *American Journal of Nursing, 49,* 496–498.
Henry, B. (1989a). Epistemological approaches to interdisciplinary inquiry for nursing administration. In B. Henry, C. Arndt, M. DiVincenti, & A. Marriner-Tomey (Eds.), *Dimensions of nursing administration* (pp. 235–246). Boston: Blackwell Scientific.
Henry, B. (1989b). The value of public administration education. *Journal of Nursing Administration, 19*(11), 4, 6, 9.
Henry, B. (1989c). The crisis in nursing administration education. *Journal of Nursing Administration, 19*(3), 6–7, 28.
Hill, B. A. (1989). The development of a master's degree program based on perceived future practice needs. *Journal of Nursing Education, 28,* 307–313.
Jennings, B. M., & Meleis, A. I. (1988). Nursing theory and administrative practice: Agenda for the 1990s. *Advances in Nursing Science, 10*(3), 56–69.
Larson, N. (1990). *MaxThink*™ [Computer Program]. Piedmont, CA: Author.
Mark, B. A., Turner, J. T., & Englebardt, S. (1990). Knowledge and skills for nurse administrators. *Nursing and Health Care, 11,* 185–189.
Marriner-Tomey, A. (1989a). Survey of theory in nursing administration textbooks. *Nursing Administration Quarterly, 13*(4), 69–70.
Marriner-Tomey, A. (1989b). Survey of doctoral programs. *Nursing Administration Quarterly, 13*(4), 67–69.
McCloskey, J. C., Gardner, D., Johnson, M., & Maas, M. (1988). What is the study of nursing service administration? *Journal of Professional Nursing, 4*(2), 92–98.
McClure, M. L. (1985). Educational preparation for nursing administration. *Nursing and Health Care, 6,* 231.
Moore, K., Biordi, D., Holm, K., & McElmurry, B. (1988). Nurse executive effectiveness. *Journal of Nursing Administration, 18*(12), 23–27.
Mullane, M. K. (1959). *Education for nursing service administration.* Battle Creek, MI: W. K. Kellogg Foundation.

Neidlinger, S. H., & Miller, M. B. (1990). Nursing care delivery systems: A nursing administrative practice perspective. *Journal of Nursing Administration, 20*(10), 43–49.

Nyberg, J. (1990). Theoretic explorations of human care and economics: Foundations of nursing administration practice. *Advances in Nursing Science, 13*(1), 74–84.

Peterson, H. E., & Gerdin-Jelger, U. (1988). *Preparing nurses for using information systems: Recommended informatics competencies* (NLN Pub. No. 14-2234). New York: National League for Nursing.

Pfoutz, S. K., Simms, L. M., & Price, S. A. (1987). Teaching and learning: Essential components of the nurse executive role. *Image: Journal of Nursing Scholarship, 19,* 138–141.

Poulin, M. A. (1979). Education for nurse administrators. *Nursing Administration Quarterly, 3*(4), 45–51.

Poulin, M. A. (1984). The nurse executive role: A structural and functional analysis. *Journal of Nursing Administration, 14*(2), 9–14.

Price, S. A. (1984). Master's programs preparing nurse administrators: What are the essential components? *Journal of Nursing Administration, 14*(1), 11–17.

Ray, M. A. (1989). The theory of bureaucratic caring for nursing practice in the organizational culture. *Nursing Administration Quarterly, 13*(2), 31–42.

Reynolds, B. J. (1987). Directors of nursing service: How well prepared are they? *Nursing Outlook, 35,* 274–287.

Scalzi, C. S., & Anderson, R. A. (1989a). Dual degree. Future preparation for nurse executives? *Journal of Nursing Administration, 19*(6), 25–29.

Scalzi, C. S., & Anderson, R. A. (1989b). Conceptual model for theory development in nursing administration. In B. Henry, C. Arndt, M. DiVincenti, & A. Marriner-Tomey (Eds.), *Dimensions of nursing administration* (pp. 137–141). Boston: Blackwell Scientific.

Schultz, P. R. (1987). When client means more than one: Extending the foundational concepts of person. *Advances in Nursing Science, 10*(1), 71–86.

Schultz, P. R., & Miller, K. L. (1990). Nursing administration research, Part one: Pluralities of persons. In J. J. Fitzpatrick, R. L. Taunton, & J. Q. Benoliel (Eds.), *Annual Review of Nursing Research, Volume 8,* (pp. 133–158). New York: Springer Publishing Co.

Simms, L. M. (1988). Education for Administration in Nursing: Preparing Nursing Administrators. *Journal of Nursing Administration, 18*(2), 4.

Simms, L. M., Price, S. A., & Pfoutz, S. K. (1985). Nurse executives: Functions and priorities. *Nursing Economics, 3,* 238–244.

Stepura, B. A., & Tilbury, M. A. (1988). An analysis of academic programs preparing nurse administrators. *Journal of Nursing Administration, 18*(5), 8.

Stevens, B. J. (1978). Education in nursing administration: Where are we and where should we be? In C. H. Slater (Ed.), *The education and roles of nursing service administrators* (pp. 21–38). Battle Creek, MI: W. K. Kellogg Foundation.

Thomas, B., Erickson, E. H., & Heick, M. (1974). Survey of nursing service administration graduates. *Nursing Outlook, 22,* 457–459.

Vance, C., & Wolf, M. S. (1986). Essential skills for nurse managers. *Journal of Nursing Administration, 16*(12), 9, 16.

Wagner, L., Henry, B., Giovinco, G., & Blanks, C. (1988). Suggestions for graduate education in nursing service administration. *Journal of Nursing Education, 27,* 210–218.

Wiley, K. (1989). Focus of research for PhD in Nursing. *Journal of Nursing Education, 28,* 190–192.

PART IV

Research on the Profession of Nursing

Chapter 10

The Staff Nurse Role

NORMA L. CHASKA
SCHOOL OF NURSING
UNIVERSITY OF SAN FRANCISCO

CONTENTS

The staff nurse role—what it is and what it is not—is a continuing problem plaguing the delivery of nursing care. The role is a particular target of concern for the 1990s because of the emphasis within the profession on differentiating levels of practice. Curtin (1990) views that it is necessary to delineate the role according to the different settings for care rather than different levels of practice within settings. As the staff nursing role becomes defined clearly within the overall system of care, the most important consideration will be the relationship aspects of the role that is, how the staff nurse interacts with other health care personnel, such as head nurses, clinical nurse, specialists, and physicians.

The initial studies concerning nursing role were conducted in the 1960s and addressed role conceptualization (Corwin, 1961; Corwin & Taves, 1962; Harrington & Theis, 1968; Kramer, 1968, 1969). Kramer (1970, 1972) and others (Benner & Kramer, 1972; Chaska, 1978; Davis & Underwood, 1976; McCloskey, 1974; Minehan, 1977; Reichow & Scott, 1976) followed in the 1970s by focusing on the functions and values, as well as the conception of the nursing role. Cantor and Mischel (1979) explored social cognition theory and focused on processing information into schemes.

The purpose of this chapter is to summarize and critique the major investigations about the staff nurse role that have been conducted in the 1980s and early 1990s. First, role reconceptualization and the frameworks that are being advocated are addressed. Findings about what staff nurses do and major issues, problems, and challenges in relation to the staff nurse role are discussed. Relationships pertinent to the role and future evolution of the role are emphasized. Finally, directions for future research are suggested.

ROLE RECONCEPTUALIZATION

Context of Practice in Organizations

There has been a diffusion of professional responsibilities and an expansion of functions and tasks for nurses functioning in the staff nurse role. For example, patient and family teaching now may be done by patient educators who are not nurses, but, on the other hand, the nurse is charged with more decision-making authority in patient care than previously (Singleton & Nail, 1984). There are efforts to maximize professional autonomy within the organizations in which staff nurses practice.

Considerable research has been focused on the role orientations of nurses in general as these orientations relate to their work and to organizational variables (Ketefian, 1985). Attitudes are thought to influence the perceptions and performance of the individual. Bureaucratic, professional, and service orientations were the basis for conceptualizing the early nursing role studies (Corwin, 1961). The bureaucratic role conception emphasizes rules and regulations within the organization, with primary loyalty to administration. The professional role conception is associated with principles and standards of a profession, with primary loyalty to the profession. The service role orientation is associated with values such as humanity, compassion, and dedication, with primary loyalty to the patient (Kinney, 1985). Corwin (1961) found that baccalaureate graduates held high professional role conceptions more frequently than did diploma graduates. The baccalaureate graduates also experienced greater conflicts between their ideal role and their view of the way they were able to enact the ideal role. Kramer (1968, 1969, 1970, 1972, 1974) examined the conflict between bureaucratic and professional orientations. She found that nurses left the profession largely because of the antithetical nature of the bureaucratic and professional role orientations. She proposed that "success" in the nursing role was dependent on the ability to integrate both orientations (Kramer, 1972, 1974).

Later, Ketefian (1981, 1985) selected moral behavior as an index of professional behavior. Moral judgments as behavior refers to the determination of right or wrong in a given situation, and the focus is on nurses' decision making and the critical and rational analyses for moral decision making. Ketefian (1985) found a positive relationship between moral behavior and professional role conception, with the latter a better predictor of moral behavior than was bureaucratic role conception.

Early conceptualizations of the nursing role did not consider an important factor that was recognized by Ketefian (1985). She suggested that certain practice settings allow greater freedom to make independent professional judgments than other settings, such as hospitals. Ketefian posited that certain organizational settings serve to reinforce rather than change the role orientation and practice of nurses (1985).

Practice setting is the key variable that must be acknowledged in reconceptualizing the nursing role. More importantly, *positions* within the setting must be defined, as the nature of a position in a bureaucracy may greatly influence role conceptualization. For example, the staff nurse role assumes that there is a position titled "staff nurse," or some similar title, in a particular institution or organization. The term conveys something more than a role. Most research on staff nurses has been focused on a generic nursing role, not necessarily linking role orientation with a particular setting. Typically, "staff nurse" is a *position* role, specific to hospital institutions acknowledging both a formal position and a nursing role within that bureaucratic setting. Recent conceptualization of a staff nurse role, then, goes beyond the orientations of the 1960s and 1970s.

Definition of Constructs

For purposes of this review, the term "staff nurse role" refers to a generalist, clinical nursing role held by a registered nurse in a first-level clinical nursing position in a hospital setting. Incorporated in the staff nurse role are orientations that may be conceptualized as bureaucratic, professional, service, or moral. These orientations were described in research conducted in the 1960s and 1970s (Ketefian, 1985; Kinney, 1985). The orientations refer, respectively, to the policies and formalized structure, such as job descriptions, inherent in bureaucratic settings that are associated with the delivery of nursing care, principles and standards of professional nursing practice, humanistic values associated with providing health and illness care, and the determination of right or wrong in nurses decisions for a given nursing care situation. More recent studies, in contrast to earlier research, have focused on a combination of orientations for complex multidimensions of the staff nurse role. Consequently, the review in this chapter includes varying dimensions and constructs of the hospital staff nurse role.

Literature Reviewed

Data bases used in searching the literature were: (a) NAHL, the on-line version of CINAHL, which is the Cumulative Index to Nursing and Allied Health Literature; (b) MEDLINE; (c) SOCA; (d) PsycLIT; and (e) Health. The first criterion for the review was that the article concern a nursing role. Within that broad criterion, articles were selected based on criteria that: (a) a generalist type of clinical nursing role was addressed, (b) the article was data based, or (c) an aspect of the research process was addressed in relation to a generalist nursing role.

An extensive review of the literature revealed 97 articles concerning the nursing role that were published from 1960 to 1990. The majority, approximately 50, that were conducted in the 1960s and 1970s were focused on one or more of 6 variables: (a) academic achievement, (b) family of origin characteristics, (c) demographic characteristics of nurses, (d) employment characteristics, (e) nursing school characteristics, and (f) nurse career behaviors. Studies conducted in the 1980s and 1990s may be classified into three broad and overlapping categories: (a) those dealing with the functions, behaviors, and qualities associated with or specific to *what* the staff nurse *does,* (b) studies from the perspective of nurses and nursing students, and (c) those focused primarily on *problems* associated with the staff nurse role. The first large category in this review focuses on dimensions of professional practice. These included studies of: (a) role orientation, (b) role stereotypes, (c) staff nurse role components, (d) staff nurse behaviors and qualities, (e) role differentiation between nurse and physician, (f) collaborative role models, (g) professional role socialization, and (h) role modeling. The second category emphasized perspectives of nurses and nursing students. The third category included studies that focused predominantly on the *problems* in: (a) role enactment, including nurse–physician interaction, role interfaces, and role strain, and (b) implications of the problems for professional practice and job satisfaction. The first two categories are addressed as "Findings: Role Explication" in this chapter. The third category is discussed predominantly in the section "Findings: Major Issues" to highlight the challenges evident in role delineation of the staff nurse. Challenges for resolution are discussed in "Directions for Future Research."

FINDINGS: ROLE EXPLICATION

Dimensions of Professional Practice

Role conceptualization underlies the delineation of the dimensions of professional practice. Ketefian (1985) found that a professional role framework was related in practice to moral behavior and to feelings of a greater degree of conflict between the professional and bureaucratic roles. She concluded that actual professional practice does not meet nurses' expectations and that bureaucratic role requirements exceed their expectations. From her findings, Ketefian suggested that education shapes the role orientation of the staff nurse.

Kinney (1985) found that masculinity–femininity attributes were more closely associated with role conceptions than with personality characteristics. The feminine attributes in her study were related to professional and service role conceptions, whereas both feminine and masculine attributes were related to bureaucratic and service orientations.

Kaler, Levy, and Schall (1989) studied the nursing role orientation of the public. They found that the traditionally held view of nurses by the public was that of a "helping" profession. Concern for others and attributes associated with femininity and nurturance were common in the stereotypes of nurses. The researchers concluded that the nursing emphasis on scholarliness has yet to be transmitted to the public; however, as Aydelotte (1987) warned, scholarliness will not happen until nurses actually are empowered with autonomy. The need for autonomy in professional practice is underscored by Kaler and colleagues' findings.

Building on the suggestions of Cantor and Mischel (1979), a number of investigations have been focused on the behaviors and qualities associated with professional practice. These include: Alexander, Weisman, and Chase (1982), Andersen (1989), Bennett (1984), Chaska (1978, 1988, 1990), Chaska, Clark, Rogers, and Deets (1990), Chaska, Clark, Rogers, and Deets (in press), Corcoran (1986), Dennis and Prescott (1985), Hendrickson and Doddato, (1989), Katzman and Roberts (1988), Katzman (1989), Norris (1989), Prescott and Bowen (1985), Prescott, Dennis, Creasia, and Bowen (1985),

Prescott, Dennis, and Jacox (1987), Raelin (1989), Rothrock (1985), Swider, McElmurry, and Yarling (1985), Tarsitano, Brophy, and Snyder (1986), and Weiss (1985).

Dennis and Prescott (1985) addressed specific qualities and behaviors associated with the professional role through the historical tie with Nightingale. Qualitative data findings from their study included such hallmarks of professional practice as genuine concern for patients, maturity, commitment, and intelligence.

Several researchers emphasized behaviors and qualities related to human values, ethics, and caring in the staff nurse role (Curtin, 1990; Norris, 1989; Reverby, 1987). Norris (1989) cautioned that conceptual definitions of such qualities of behaviors as caring are insufficient, and that operational definitions stated in behavioral terms are essential for testing, measurement, and evaluation to occur.

Other researchers identified variables related to autonomy in professional nursing practice. Alexander and colleagues (1982) analyzed the organizational determinants of staff nurses' perceived autonomy. They found five variables that significantly predicted perceived autonomy: (a) baccalaureate education, (b) internal locus of control, (c) primary nursing as a method of organizing nursing care, (d) the staff nurse's attitudes toward her or his head nurse's leadership style and responsiveness, and (e) the adequacy of professional time. The latter was defined as time to devote to professional development. The common belief that special care units attract nurses who have greater personal control beliefs and thus are likely to report greater levels of work-related autonomy was not supported. Nurses in their first positions, those who rotated shifts on special units, and nurses who positively evaluated their head nurse reported the highest perceived autonomy. The findings of Alexander et al. indicated that nurses' perceptions of autonomy were influenced by both personal characteristics of the nurse and structural features of the units.

Raelin (1989) explored issues related to the administrative autonomy of unit managers and the operational autonomy of professionals such as primary care staff nurses. He concluded that there are situations in which nonmanagerial professionals should be granted administrative and strategic autonomy to control or coordinate their work and times when managers ought to be granted operational autonomy to control the means, conditions, processes, and procedures of work. Based on data from intensive interviews, he categorized the conditions under which the traditional view of autonomy might be reversed. A study of Singleton and Nail (1984) indicated that autonomous practice is dependent on the structure of a given institution.

Another dimension of professional practice concerns behaviors and qualities related to decision making. Swider et al. (1985) examined decisions made by senior nursing students (potential first-level staff nurses) in response to a hypothetical ethical dilemma posed in a hospital setting. In exploring the process of decision making, they found that students first sought to work within the system for resolving dilemmas, that is, they chose a bureaucratic-centered approach.

Prescott and colleagues (1987), in interviews with staff nurses and physicians, explored clinical decision making as part of a larger study. From a content analysis of data, they inferred satisfaction among staff nurses in relation to making clinical decisions under four conditions: when the nurses (a) had input into the decision-making process, (b) believed they had a certain amount of decision-making freedom, (c) thought that the satisfaction or dissatisfaction of nurses with their roles in clinical decision making was not a factor in nursing vacancy and turnover, and when (d) physicians listened to their input and considered their suggestions.

In the Prescott et al. (1987) study, two ways of categorizing decisions emerged from analysis of the nature of the staff nurse role: (a) decisions nurses *can* make, and (b) those they *want* to make. The broad domain for decisions included: (a) patient assessment, (b) patient care, for example, drawing blood gases, inserting nasogastric tube, (c) giving medications, (d) physical care, such as changing a diet, applying restraints, and (e) patient teaching. The major difference, between physicians' and nurses' descriptions about decision making was their interpretation of nurses' involvement in what comprises a decision. Physicians viewed the last stage, selecting a course of action, as decision making, whereas nurses viewed earlier stages of the process, such as collecting information and identifying problems, as decision making. In the former situation, physicians saw themselves as making all the decisions, with nurses assisting and having little authority; with the latter view, nurses were satisfied with their level of involvement given that physicians valued their input.

Corcoran (1986) investigated task complexity as a factor in decision making by staff nurses. She found that the cognitive processing of decisions in planning care was contingent on demands of task domains within a complex environment. For example, inexperienced staff nurses focused on a single intervention to alleviate a problem, such as pain, rather than developing a broad view of the patient.

Building from previous research and the literature, Chaska (1978, 1988, 1990) and colleagues (1990, in press) identified behaviors and qualities associated with the staff nurse role. She found that behavior among professionals was shaped by the demands of others and the environment, sanctions, and the person's own conceptions of what her or his role is or should be.

In Chaska's studies, independent scales were developed to measure nurses' and physicians' expectations and perceptions of the staff nurse role in relation to 11 factors. These factors included nursing role activities, organizational influences, and physican role activities in relation to the staff nurse role. The nursing role scales concerned: (a) patient assessment, (b) medical-technical tasks, (c) nursing judgment, (d) registered nurse (RN) communication, (e) liaison activities, (f) current role beliefs for RNs, and (g) collaboration functions. The physician role scales pertained to: (a) communication, (b) legal responsibilities, and (c) understanding of the RN role. Differences were found in expectations and perceptions of role behavior between nurses and physicians (Chaska et al., 1990), particularly in relation to the independent, dependent, and interdependent aspects of the staff nurse role.

Role Components: Functions and Tasks

Hendrickson and Doddato (1989) identified the components of the staff nurse role as viewed by nurses. Questionnaires were distributed to 313 staff nurses in randomly selected nursing units. Professional nursing components were found to include collaborative activities and "higher order" (p. 281) functional tasks. Examples of the former included developing care plans and participating in nursing and medical rounds. The latter tasks encompassed documenting care and preparing and giving medications.

Time limitations are a factor in care, requiring priorities to be set among competing tasks, and Hendrickson and Doddato (1989) also addressed that issue. Although the staff nurses in their study indicated that they wanted to spend more time on and increase collaborative activities, those aspects of their role were the first to be neglected. Staff nurses made certain that the higher-order functional tasks were carried out first and would do these tasks if necessary when time was short rather than perform professional activities. For example, if no one else was available to transport or weigh a patient, change linens, or tidy a patient's room, the nurse did them.

Additional components of the staff nurse role have been identified by a number of other investigators (Alexander et al., 1982; Corcoran, 1986; Roberts, 1983; Tarsitano et al., 1986; Taunton & Otteman, 1986; Wolf, 1986, 1989). For example, Andersen (1989) and Rothrock (1985) addressed elements of being a nurse advocate and patient advocate as part of the staff nurse role. Rothrock (1985) and Ketefian (1981, 1985) further discussed role aspects involving ethics and moral reasoning. Bennett (1984) pointed out some of the legal fundamentals in the role. Finally, Masson (1985) concluded that the principal function of nurses is healing; she described nursing and medicine as complementary modes toward this end.

Although Tarsitano and colleagues (1986) investigated primarily the clinical specialist role, from their research findings components of the first-level clinical nursing position can be inferred. Professional clinical practice activities in providing direct patient care were clearly defined in their study. These included such functions as: (a) assessment, (b) establishing nursing diagnoses, (c) patient teaching, (d) decision making, and (e) assisting or collaborating with other health professionals in providing care. These clinical practice elements also were cited in the research findings related to the role functions previously reviewed.

The following are examples of other studies related to role components. Planning and assessment were suggested by Corcoran (1986) as part of decision making, and the latter also was explored by Swider and colleagues (1985). Autonomy was identified as an integral component of the staff nurse role by Alexander et al. (1982). Wolf (1989) identified some of the physical, interpersonal communication, and cognitive tasks of the role.

Chaska and colleagues' (1990) study provides a useful compendium of staff nurse role components because this study incorporated all of the role orientations and almost all of the functions previously suggested by other researchers. As mentioned earlier, Chaska developed 11 scales to measure 7 types of nursing behaviors, 3 categories of physician behaviors, and organizational influence. One of the scales, Current Role, measures the integration of the different role orientations. The remaining 10 scales address functions addressed by Alexander et al. (1982), Corcoran (1986), Hendrickson and Doddato (1989), Ketefian (1985), McLain (1988), Prescott et al. (1987), Singleton and Nail (1984), Swider et al. (1985), Tarsitano et al. (1986), Weiss (1983, 1985), Weiss and Davis (1985), and Wolf (1989).

Role Differentiation

The lack of consensus regarding the staff nurse role as differentiated from medical practice and shared areas of common practice contributes to pseudo-collaboration in providing care (Weiss, 1983). In Weiss's study of 417 specific role behaviors, respondents viewed the majority of health care activities as being overlapping or as shared responsibilities of both nurse and physician. Weiss further found that in shared areas of common practice, physicians were rated higher for the degree to which activities and role behaviors were designated as responsibilities within the domain of medical practice rather than nursing. No single behavior was identified as being a unique nursing responsibility.

Later, Weiss and Davis (1985) attempted to clarify mutual responsibilities in practice through the development of collaborative practice scales. However, the relatively low validity and reliability of their scales provide rationale for continued refinement of the measures. Further testing of the scales with larger samples from various care settings is indicated. In another study, Weiss (1985) found that ongoing discourse (between nurses and physicians) enhanced traditional beliefs about the authority and power of the physician rather than fostering collaborative values.

McLain (1988) investigated role differentiation in terms of nurses' and physicians' failure to collaborate appropriately. She found that distorted communication and nonmeaningful interactions were promoted by both nurses and physicians. Based on her findings it is suggested that underlying values and beliefs determine the nature of collaborative practice.

Congruity–Discrepancy with Expectations

Congruity among job requirements, expectations, and individual needs and abilities were shown in the 1970s to increase job satisfaction (Kramer & Schmalenberg, 1979) and to be related to professional and organizational socialization (Forrester, 1988). Discrepancy in the staff nurse role refers to disparity between idealized role conceptions or expectations and perceptions of actual role enactment (Forrester, 1988).

Due to the findings of recent studies conducted by Oechsle and Landry (1987) and by Forrester (1988), these researchers suggested a need to modify beliefs about expectations and perceptions as related to role discrepancies. Oechsle and Landry (1987) attempted to develop a measure for congruity of expectations. They found congruity between prior expectations and perceptions of the work situation in their respondents, unaffected by age and prior work experience of the staff nurses.

Forrester (1988) examined the relationship between sex role identity and perceptions of nurse role discrepancy among staff nurses. He found that regardless of sex role identity, staff nurses continued to have significant levels of role discrepancy. Further, staff nurses viewed professional and service-oriented values as existing less and bureaucratic values or situations as existing more than they ideally thought they should. Additionally, special-care hospital unit staff nurses perceive more discrepancy between service and bureaucratic expectations than nurses practicing in general hospital units.

Chaska and colleagues (in press) suggested two other factors that may influence congruity–discrepancy with expectations. They indicated that, according to their data, staff nurses may be influenced more by the expectations of physicians than by those of nurses in relation to professional practice. Although nurses had higher expectations than physicians for independent role functions, physicians and nurses agreed as regarding the extent to which these functions were conducted and had low perception scores for those behaviors. Confusion among the nurses and physicians about the initial education nursing programs was a possible source for misunderstanding role preparation and expectations.

Role Models

The dilemma of role adjustment for new staff nurses has been addressed by numerous investigators (Green, 1988; Little & Brian, 1982; Lynn, McCain, & Boss, 1989; Olsson & Gullberg, 1988; Talotta, 1990; Williams, 1989). Predominantly, role modeling was examined as a means for professional socialization, which is considered a crucial issue in nursing today (McCain, 1985).

Green (1988) found that: (a) faculty role models are shortly replaced by work-related models for new graduates, (b) clinical experience-performance is the most important role model characteristic, and (c) role perception orientations are professional prior to graduation but change to a more bureaucratic orientation after exposure to work-related models. Buckenham (1988) examined the importance of five role functions (administrative, clinical, interpersonal, management, and teaching) held by nursing students as compared with staff nurses. Whereas first-year students differed significantly from the staff nurse, third-year students were found to have similar expectations. The finding that management functions increased and clinical activities decreased in importance was attributed to the influence of role models.

Little and Brian (1982) found that most nurses were affected by additional education, but not in the same way. They investigated changes in role conceptions as nurses advanced from an initial 2-year or 3-year nursing program through a baccalaureate degree. State of readiness and receptivity were suggested as influencing variables.

The process of professional socialization, that is, the formation and internalization of a professional identity congruent with the professional role, was the focus of a longitudinal study conducted by Lynn and colleagues (1989). The primary instrument used was the Nurses' Professional Orientation Scale (NPOS) (Crocker & Brodie, 1974), which measures the congruence between students' perceptions and faculty members' conceptions of the professional nursing role. It is a 59-item rating scale composed of a variety of attitudinal and behavioral attributes of nurses. The alpha estimates for internal consistency have ranged from .88 to .92 in previous studies. For this study, the reliability was .79, believed to be due to a more homogeneous group of study subjects. Lynn and colleagues (1989) found no change in the registered nurse–bachelor of nursing science (RN/BSN) students' professional orientation during the time of their baccalaureate education, while the generic students changed to be more in alignment with their faculty than did the RN/BSN students. The significant differences found between RN/BSN and generic (BSN students not yet licensed as RNs) graduates raise serious questions. What effect is there on education outcomes and patient care when the RN/BSN students do not share similar views of nursing with the generic student? Should research be focused on attitude conversion rather than professional socialization?

FINDINGS: MAJOR ISSUES

Barriers to Role Enactment

Three dominant problems related to role enactment are: (a) conflicts in physician and nurse interaction, (b) role interfaces, and (c) role strain. The first two issues have been extensively investigated (Hodes & Van Combrugghe, 1990; Katzman, 1989; Katzman & Roberts, 1988; McLain, 1988; Mechanic & Aiken, 1982; Prescott & Bowen, 1985; Stein, Watts, & Howell, 1990). Lack of mutual understanding regarding the problems each group faces is believed to be a key factor (Mechanic & Aiken, 1982). Lack of collaboration (McLain, 1988) and lack of basic interaction (Katzman & Roberts, 1988) were found to be other contributing variables. Relationships were found to be more important than internal or external work rewards according to a study by Williams (1990).

Katzman (1989) reported that differences between nurses' and physicians' views about current and ideal authority of nurses is a significant variable. Prescott and Bowen (1985) examined the areas of conflict and found that disagreements centered predominantly on patient care, and variability in nurses' competence was an issue. Stein and colleagues (1990) suggested from their findings that change in the physician–nurse relationship is beneficial for mutually interdependent roles.

Tarsitano et al. (1986) found that lack of congruence in role expectations, particularly between professional groups, contributed to role strain. Ward (1986) defined role strain within the context of role stress and related it to job dissatisfaction.

Implications of the Major Issues

The inability of staff nurses to practice their role as they envision it may lead to dissatisfaction in their job, decreased organizational commitment, and decreased professionalism (McCloskey & McCain, 1987). Restructuring the work place for new practice models in care delivery is suggested by the research findings of Minnick, Roberts, Curran, and Ginzberg (1989). McCloskey and McCain (1987) concluded that employers need to assess the initial expectations of new nurses, then meet more of their expectations or help nurses to form more realistic ones.

Weiss (1983) found two problems related to ambiguity in role enactment: (a) lack of clarity within the profession of nursing about the competencies specific to the discipline of nursing, and (b) in continuing public image of nurses as only physician extenders. Equally problematic may be the attitudes and behaviors of nurses themselves. The understanding that many nurses see no role domain exclusively as their own was supported through research conducted by Weiss and Remen (1983).

CRITIQUE

Methodologic and Measurement Concerns

There are several points to be made regarding research about the staff nurse role. Practice setting is a variable that was acknowledged insufficiently in the investigations that were reviewed. Structural complexity of the staff nurse work role is a critical factor in role explication that varies with settings. For example, in a hospital the role of a general staff nurse in intensive care units may be different from the role on general medical-surgical nursing units. The effect of complex, highly skilled, technical role behaviors required in certain types of nursing units at the expense of integrating, expressive, service role type of behaviors needs exploration. Clinical area of practice, worksite, or unit assignment were the subjects of few studies. According to Schwirian (1981), investigators most often have treated the placement of staff nurses and their roles like "interchangeable checkers."

A systematic comparison of findings from the studies reviewed was difficult given the variance in design, sampling procedures, sample size, type of data (qualitative versus quantitative), variables studied, measurement, and data analysis. Most studies in this review dealt with academic achievement, nurses' personal characteristics, and programs of nursing students as predictors of performance, with a lesser number concerned with employment characteristics. Few studies have been conducted from the perspective of staff nurses themselves, as opposed to the perspective of those who employ nurses.

There were great differences in the analytical techniques used in the investigations reviewed. Nonparametric statistics were most frequently used, followed by parametric techniques. Because the staff nurse role is multidimensional, more information could have been obtained by applying multivariate techniques.

Schwirian (1981) suggested that factor analysis and factor mapping, to identify the underlying structure of specific indicators related to a model of nursing performance or to develop summary indexes of the various categories of variables in a causal network, should be the analytical techniques used in research of the 1980s and 1990s. These techniques were rarely used in the studies reviewed.

Validity and reliability for the numerous investigative scales developed are major issues, with the internal consistency reliabilities of subscales problematic. Ketefian (1985) cited the problem of internal consistency reliability in role studies.

Role Explication Concerns

Findings from research concerning the dimensions and determinants of professional practice were inconclusive. The major contributions of the studies reviewed may be to: (a) affirm that the staff nurse role is unclear, (b) provide documentation regarding variables that may influence the role, (c) suggest problematic areas for further investigation, (d) support the need for consistent expectations in behaviors for professional practice, and (e) further clarify major components of the staff nurse role.

It was difficult to compare components of the staff nurse role across the studies reviewed. Most studies were conducted under severe constraints. There was a paucity of research encompassing all of the major factors that were suggested as significant for the staff nurse role. Therefore, consensus regarding the components is still lacking.

Additional questions related to the interdependence between nursing and medicine need to be addressed. These include: (a) how and to what extent is true equality in collaboration a realistic goal? and (b) what factors influence equality in collaboration?

The factors that significantly influence congruity–discrepancy with expectations have not been clearly delineated. There was evidence that multiple variables are related, as previously was suggested between mutliple role dimensions and the structural setting for practice. Differences in role expectations were shown to occur, but few such studies were conducted. The influence of differing philosophies in educational programs on ideal role models in practice should be further studied.

Role modeling and professional socialization in nursing were insufficiently studied areas. Few instruments have been developed to measure the concepts and processes. The role conceptions of role models were virtually unknown. The work experience of staff nurses as part of an ongoing professional socialization process was a neglected phenomenon for inquiry.

Interprofessional conflicts between nurses and physicians are part of nursing's history. More recent research findings not only implicated interprofessional conflicts but suggested overlapping areas of responsibility and role strain as barriers to professional nursing practice and as problems in health care.

Methodologic issues, such as arbitrary choice of an endpoint for socialization and the lack of predictive validity of instruments, were problematic in the studies of professional socialization. An additional concern was the focus of socialization research, such as in translating attitudinal changes into behavioral role changes.

DIRECTIONS FOR FUTURE RESEARCH

Research Areas

Research is needed to identify the relationships among role conceptions and components of the staff nurse role. Factors that lead to bureaucratic role conceptions, unsatisfactory work environments, and tendencies to hold rigidly to rules and regulations need to be further identified. Specific factors that should be examined, for their effects on the staff nurse role are: (a) specialty versus general units, (b) structural design of units, (c) situational differences, such as emergency versus nonemergency, and (d) organizational variables in the practice setting.

Research needs to be designed to test, increase, and evaluate: (a) the understanding of the staff nurse role, (b) professional role development and socialization, (c) collaboration, and (d) negotiation and resolution of staff nurse role conflict. Collaborative professional governance in hospitals should be tested.

Experimental testing of structures that may be most supportive for staff nurse role enactment should be conducted. The use of assistants in providing care, such as auxiliaries cited by Sovie (1989), require further investigation. The structure and process of resolving organizational constraints affecting role behavior is a valuable area for exploration. Munro (1983) has suggested that areas of satisfaction or dissatisfaction specific to the staff nurse role be defined and addressed through research.

Finally, patient outcomes should be the primary concern in staff nurse role delineation. The purpose of defining high-level professional behaviors is to provide better patient care. That goal must be re-affirmed consciously and continuously. Through role delineation, expectations for behaviors may be more clearly defined between and among health professionals. In particular, physicians and nurses working together with explicitly understood roles may offer a higher quality of care than by either professional workers alone.

Methodologies

Sophisticated approaches are needed in future research on the staff nurse role, including the use of experimental designs and both qualitative and quantitative methods in the same study. Replication of previous research, particularly those studies utilizing multivariate analysis, would be of value. Larger, randomly selected samples from various groups and organizational settings are needed as are multisite studies. More instruments need to be developed and tested to measure the staff nurse role. Finally, effort is needed to design studies whereby findings can be compared and pooled for meta-analysis purposes.

In the research reviewed for this chapter, multivariate analytical techniques were used in few studies (Alexander et al., 1982; Chaska et al., 1990; Forrester, 1988; Kinney, 1985; Oechsle and Landry, 1987; Prescott et al., 1987; Swider et al., 1985; Tarsitano et al., 1986; Weiss, 1983, 1985; Weiss & Davis, 1985). To explain differences in study findings, questions must be asked about other variables not included and about whether measurement error could be masking certain factors and relationships. Although results of the research reviewed are encouraging, for the foregoing reasons the findings are not generalizable. There is need for replication of some previous studies, for use of additional methods, and for identification of further questions and factors concerning the staff nurse role. This review of research has demonstrated the need for further communication and consensus regarding the role, scope, and conditions of professional staff nurse practice.

REFERENCES

Alexander, C. S., Weisman, C. S., & Chase, G. A. (1982). Determinants of staff nurses' perceptions of autonomy within different clinical contexts. *Nursing Research, 31*, 48–52.

Andersen, S. L. (1989). The nurse advocate project: A strategy to retain new graduates. *Journal of Nursing Administration, 19*(12), 22–26.

Aydelotte, M. K. (1987). The changing image of the nurse [Review of The changing image of the nurse]. *Image: Journal of Nursing Scholarship, 19*, 213–214.

Benner, P., & Kramer, M. (1972). Role conceptions and integrative role behavior of nurses in special care and regular hospital nursing units. *Nursing Research, 21*, 20–29.

Bennett, H. M. (1984). Good nursing practice. *Critical Care Nurse*, 68–69.

Buckenham, M. A. (1988). Student nurse perception of staff nurse role. *Journal of Advanced Nursing, 13*, 662–670.

Cantor, N., & Mischel, W. (1979). Prototypes in person perception. *Advances in Experimental Social Psychology, 12*, 3–52.

Chaska, N. (1978). Status consistency and nurses' expectations and perceptions of role performance. *Nursing Research, 27*, 356–364.

Chaska, N. (1988). Expectations and perceptions of staff nurses role performance among nurses and physicians. (Unpublished report for Methodist Hospital of Indiana, Inc., Indianapolis, IN.)

Chaska, N. (1990). Expectations and perceptions of staff nurses performance among nurses. (Unpublished report for Beth Israel Hospital, Boston, MA.)

Chaska, N., Clark, D., Rogers, S. R., & Deets, C. A. (1990). Nurses' and physicians' expectations and perceptions of staff nurse role performance as influenced by status consistency. In N. Chaska (Ed.), (1990), *The nursing profession: Turning points* (pp. 289–303). St. Louis: Mosby.

Chaska, N., Clark, D., Rogers, S. R., & Deets, C. A. (In press). Differences between nurses' and physicians' expectations and exceptions of staff nurse role performance. *Research in Nursing and Health.*

Corcoran, S. A. (1986). Task complexity and nursing expertise as factors in decision making. *Nursing Research, 35,* 107–112.

Corwin, R. G. (1961). The professional employee: A study of conflict in nursing roles. *American Journal of Sociology, 66,* 604–615.

Corwin, R. G., & Taves, M. J. (1962). Some concomitants of bureaucratic and professional conceptions of nursing role. *Nursing Research, 11,* 223–227.

Crocker, L. M., & Brodie, B. J. (1974). Development of a scale to assess student nurses' views of the professional nursing role. *Journal of Applied Psychology, 59,* 232–235.

Curtin, L. L. (1990). Designing new roles: Nursing in the '90s and beyond. *Nursing Management, 21*(2), 7–9.

Davis, A. J., & Underwood, P. (1976). Role, function, and decision making in community mental health. *Nursing Research, 25,* 256–258.

Dennis, K. E., & Prescott, P. A. (1985). Florence Nightingale: Yesterday, today, and tomorrow. *Advances in Nursing Science, 7,* 66–81.

Forrester, D. A. (1988). Sex role identity and perceptions of nurse role discrepancy. *Western Journal of Nursing Research, 10,* 600–612.

Green, G. J. (1988). Relationships between role models and role perceptions of new graduate nurses. *Nursing Research, 37,* 245–248.

Harrington, H. A., & Theis, E. C. (1968). Institutional factors perceived by baccalaureate graduates as influencing their performance as staff nurses. *Nursing Research, 17,* 228–235.

Hendrickson, G., & Doddato, T. M. (1989). Setting priorities during the shortage. *Nursing Outlook, 37,* 280–284.

Hodes, J. R., & Van Crombrugghe, P. (1990). Nurse-physician relationships. *Nursing Management, 21,* 85–89.

Kaler, S. R., Levy, D. A., & Schall, M. (1989). Stereotypes of professional roles. *Image: Journal of Nursing Scholarship, 21,* 85–89.

Katzman, E. M. (1989). Nurses' and physicians' perceptions of nursing authority. *Journal of Professional Nursing, 5,* 208–214.

Katzman, E. M., & Roberts, J. (1988). Nurse-physician conflicts as barriers to the enactment of nursing roles. *Western Journal of Nursing Research, 10,* 576–590.

Ketefian, S. (1981). Moral reasoning and moral behavior among selected groups of practicing nurses. *Nursing Research, 30,* 171–176.

Ketefian, S. (1985). Professional and bureaucratic role conceptions and moral behavior among nurses. *Nursing Research, 34,* 248–253.

Kinney, C. K. D. (1985). A re-examination of nursing role conceptions. *Nursing Research, 34,* 170–176.

Kramer, M. (1968). Role models, role conceptions and role deprivation. *Nursing Research, 17,* 115–120.
Kramer, M. (1969). Collegiate graduate nurses in medical center hospitals: Mutual challenge of duel. *Nursing Research, 18,* 196–210.
Kramer, M. (1970). Role conception of baccalaureate nurses and success in hospital nursing. *Nursing Research, 19,* 428–439.
Kramer, M. (1972). Professional-bureaucratic conflict and integrative role behaviors. In M. Batey (Ed.), *Communicating nursing research: Is the gap being bridged?* (pp. 56–71). Boulder, CO: Western Interstate Commission for Higher Education.
Kramer, M. (1974). *Reality shock: Why some nurses leave nursing*. St. Louis: Mosby.
Kramer, M., & Schmalenberg, C. (1979). *Coping with reality shock: The voices of experience*. Wakefield, MA: Contemporary Publishing.
Little, M., & Brian, S. (1982). The challengers, interactors, and mainstreamers: Second step education and nursing roles. *Nursing Research, 31,* 239–245.
Lynn, M. R., McCain, N. L., & Boss, B. J. (1989). Socialization of R.N. To B.S.N. *Image: Journal of Nursing Scholarship, 21,* 232.
Masson, V. (1985). Nurses and doctors as healers. *Nursing Outlook, 33,* 70–73.
McCain, N. L. (1985). A test of Cohen's development model for professional socialization with baccalaureate nursing students. *Journal of Nursing Education, 24,* 180–186.
McCloskey, J. (1974). Influence of rewards and incentives on staff nurse turnover rate. *Nursing Research, 14,* 341–344.
McCloskey, J. C., & McCain, B. E. (1987). Satisfaction, commitment and professionalism of newly employed nurses. *Image: Journal of Nursing Scholarship, 19,* 20–24.
McLain, B. R. (1988). Collaborative practice: A critical theory perspective. *Research in Nursing & Health, 11,* 391–398.
Mechanic, D., & Aiken, L. H. (1982). A cooperative agenda for medicine and nursing. *New England Journal of Medicine, 307,* 747–750.
Minehan, P. (1977). Nurse role conception. *Nursing Research, 6,* 374–379.
Minnick, A., Roberts, M. J., Curran, C. R., & Ginzberg, E. (1989). What do nurses want? Priorities for action. *Nursing Outlook, 37,* 214–218.
Munro, B. H. (1983). Job satisfaction among recent graduates of schools of nursing. *Nursing Research, 31,* 350–355.
Norris, C. M. (1989). To care or not care—Questions! Questions! *Nursing & Health Care, 10,* 545–550.
Oechsle, L. H., & Landry, R. G. (1987). Congruity between role expectations and actual work experience. A study of recently employed registered nurses. *Western Journal of Nursing Research, 9,* 555–557.
Olsson, H. M., & Gullberg, M. T. (1988). Nursing education and importance of professional status in nurse role. Expectations and knowledge of the nurse role. *International Journal of Nursing Studies, 25,* 287–293.
Prescott, P. A., & Bowen, S. A. (1985). Physician-nurse relationships. *Annals of Internal Medicine, 103,* 127–133.
Prescott, P. A., Dennis, K. E., Creasia, J. L., & Bowen, S. A. (1985). Nursing shortage in transition. *Image: Journal of Nursing Scholarship, 19,* 56–62.
Prescott, P. A., Dennis, K. E., & Jacox, A. K. (1987). Clinical decision making of staff nurses. *Image: Journal of Nursing Scholarship, 19,* 56–62.

Raelin, J. A. (1989). An anatomy of autonomy: Managing professionals. *The Academy of Management Executive, 3,* 216–227.
Reichow, R. W., & Scott, R. E. (1976). Study compares graduates of two-, three-, and four-year programs. *Hospitals, 50,* 95–97, 100.
Reverby, S. (1987). A caring dilemma: Womanhood and nursing in historical perspective. *Nursing Research, 36,* 5–11.
Roberts, S. J., (1983). Oppressed group behavior: Implications for nursing. *Advances in Nursing Science, 5*(4), 21–30.
Rothrock, J. C. (1985). Nurses belong at the table of the ethics committee. *AORN Journal, 41,* 527–528.
Schwirian, P. M. (1981). Toward an explanatory model of nursing performance. *Nursing Research, 30,* 247–253.
Singleton, E. K., & Nail, F. C. (1984). Role clarification: A prerequisite to autonomy. *The Journal of Nursing Administration, 14*(10), 17–22.
Sovie, M. D. (1989). Clinical nursing practices and patient outcomes: Evaluation, evolution, and revolution. *Nursing Economics, 7,* 79–85.
Stein, L. I., Watts, D. T., & Howell, T. (1990). The doctor-nurse game revisited. *New England Journal of Medicine, 322,* 546–549.
Swider, S. M., McElmurry, B. J., & Yarling, R. R. (1985). Ethical decision making in a bureaucratic context by senior nursing students. *Nursing Research, 34,* 108–112.
Talotta, D. (1990). Role conceptions and professional role discrepancy among baccalaureate nursing students employed as nurse's aides. *Image: Journal of Nursing Scholarship, 22,* 111–115.
Tarsitano, B. J., Brophy, E. B., & Snyder, D. J. (1986). A demystification of the clinical nurse specialist role: Perceptions of clinical nurse specialists and nurse administrators. *Journal of Nursing Education, 25,* 4–9.
Taunton, R., & Otteman, D. (1986). The multiple dimensions of staff nurse role conceptions. *Journal of Nursing Administration, 16*(10), 31–37.
Ward, C. R. (1986). The meaning of role strain. *Advances in Nursing Science, 8*(2), 39–49.
Weiss, S. J. (1983). Role differentiation between nurse and physician: Implications for nursing. *Research in Nursing & Health, 8,* 49–59.
Weiss, S. J. (1985). The influence of discourse on collaboration among nurses, physicians, and consumers. *Research in Nursing & Health, 8,* 49–59.
Weiss, S. J., & Davis, H. P. (1985). Validity and reliability of the collaborative practice scales. *Nursing Research, 34,* 299–305.
Weiss, S., & Remen, N. (1983). Self-limiting patterns of nursing behavior within a tripartite context involving consumers and physicians. *Western Journal of Nursing Research, 5,* 77–89.
Williams, C. (1990). Job satisfaction: Comparing CC and med/surg nurses. *Nursing Management, 21*(7), 104A–104H.
Williams, M. D. (1989). Professional socialization: One perspective on the RN-BSN experience. *Florida Nursing Review, 3*(2), 8–14.
Wolf, Z. R. (1986). *Nurses' work: The sacred and the profane*. Philadelphia: University of Pennsylvania.
Wolf, Z. R. (1989). Uncovering the hidden work of nursing. *Nursing & Health Care, 10,* 463–467.

PART V

Other Research

Chapter 11

International Nursing Research

BEVERLY M. HENRY
COLLEGE OF NURSING
UNIVERSITY OF ILLINOIS AT CHICAGO

JEAN M. NAGELKERK
DEPARTMENT OF NURSING
UNIVERSITY OF TAMPA

CONTENTS

This review is divided into three sections focusing on international nursing research for clinical care, education, and administration. In each section the discussions are framed in terms of the following questions: What problems are being addressed? Why are the problems significant in the context of science and nursing? What methodologies are used and how rigorous is the research? What is the social benefit of the work including its contribution to international understanding? "International nursing research" has been defined broadly as: (a) scientific work conducted worldwide, (b) addressing problems in clinical nursing, nursing education, or nursing administration, and (c) using the methodologies of description, hypothesis-testing, program evaluation, policy research, or diffusion of knowledge. The review is limited to studies reported in English-language publications and conducted in countries other than the United States.

THE SIGNIFICANCE OF INTERNATIONAL NURSING RESEARCH

The Forty-second World Health Assembly urged Member States and requested the Director General of the World Health Organization (WHO) to promote and support the education of nurses, including training in research methodology, to increase nurses' participation in health research programs and the health-for-all strategy (World Health Assembly [WHA], 1989). Studies are needed that reorient the practice, education, and administration of nursing to ensure that nurses participate in developing national health care strategies and in strengthening the provision of primary health care and care at all levels (WHA, 1989). Studies are needed that are focused on health promotion and disease prevention, including analyses of the cost and benefits of care, especially for the aged, for safe motherhood interventions, and the AIDS pandemic (Hankins, 1990).

Throughout the world, research by nurses is essential in the quest for new knowledge and new approaches to cost-effective care. Research training is necessary for analysis not only of the health problems commonly found in the industrialized nations—cancer, heart disease, and diabetes—but also of diseases linked to unclean water including malaria, typhoid, and filariasis. Approximately one-third of the world's population is deprived of safe drinking water (Sivard, 1989). Nurses with scientific training also are needed to identify the most significant health care needs, design and implement practical educative and administrative interventions in the communities where the problems exist, and then compare the results to those in other communities and countries (Holleran, 1988; WHO, 1984, 1987).

THE REVIEW PROCEDURE

Research published in nursing journals between 1985 and 1989 was reviewed. Two computer searches were done through the Cumulative Index to Nursing and Allied Health Literature (CINAHL) and the Medical Literature Analysis and Retrieval System on Line (MEDLINE) using the terms "international," "cross-national," and "multi-national." There were 461 research reports selected from nine journals: the *Australian Journal of Advanced Nursing* (n = 45), *Canadian Journal of Nursing Research* (n = 74), *International Journal of Nursing Studies* (n = 71), *International Nursing Review* (n = 11), *Image: Journal of Nursing Scholarship* (n = 5), *Journal of Advanced Nursing* (n = 192), *Nursing Research* (n = 2), *Scandinavian Journal of Caring Sciences* (n

= 53), and the *Western Journal of Nursing Research* (n = 8). To broaden the analysis, 88 studies in the 1980, 1984, 1985, and 1989 proceedings of the Workgroup of European Nurse Researchers were also included for a total of 549 research reports. Each report was analyzed using a 36-item tool designed by the authors to describe the problems, methodologies, scientific merit, social benefit, and authorship.

To strengthen the conceptual analysis, all nurses' associations holding membership in the International Council of Nurses were sent a letter with queries about nursing research activities; 24 responded. Descriptions of research activities and sample publications were returned from 21 countries in five of the six world regions as designated by the World Health Organization. The regions and countries included: *Africa*—Zambia; the *Americas*—Canada, United States; *Europe*—Austria, Belgium, Denmark, Finland, Germany, Greece, Israel, Norway, Sweden, Switzerland, the United Kingdom; *South-East Asia*—India, Nepal, Thailand; *Western Pacific*—Australia, Japan, Korea, the Philippines. A relatively large sample of research reports was selected and a variety of documents, correspondence, and printed materials was used to ensure a degree of data-related validity.

The authors are aware of some of the problems with studies called "international" (Scheuch, 1990). Cross-cultural comparisons are sometimes considered more scholarly (Teune, 1990). A comprehensive approach was selected because it seemed relevant to the future of nursing science, the substantive sharing of information about primary health care and care at all levels, and improved methodologic training. Throughout the review, studies have been highlighted because of their strengths and also to improve understanding of nursing research in as broad a range of national contexts as possible. The criteria used to judge the strength of the research were scientific merit and social benefit.

ANALYSIS OF INTERNATIONAL RESEARCH IN NURSING

The research problems in the studies were identified, with approximately 50% pertaining to clinical practice, 25% to nursing education, and 15% to nursing administration. The remaining related to the nursing profession. Three-quarters of the studies were descriptive, about 14% were hypothesis-testing, 6% were program evaluations, and the few remaining were analyses of diffusion or policy research. Three-fourths of the studies were cross-sectional, and a nurse was the first author in three-quarters of the publications. In each of the sections described below, examples of the studies reviewed are included for illustrative purposes.

Clinical Nursing Research

Of the 549 research reports, 305 were categorized as clinical nursing research. The main themes were nursing assessment, interventions, and client education; perceptions and attitudes of caregivers and clients; or evaluation of the quality of care. Comparatively few studies were found focusing on problems related to communicable disease. More than half the clinical studies were also grouped as pertaining to adult health and gerontology, about one-third as maternal–child health, and the few remaining as mental health or communicable diseases. Two-thirds were exploratory or descriptive, and the remaining were either experimental or methodologic. Convenience samples were reported in about half the studies. Random selection was reported in only 15. Reliability and validity were not consistently reported.

Nursing Assessment, Interventions, and Client Education. The major causes of death and disability for people in industrialized countries are the health problems associated with cardiovascular disease, cancer, and degenerative maladies. A number of significant exploratory studies addressing these health problems have been reported in the international literature. In Canada, Ford (1989), interested in evaluating the psychosocial aspects of cardiac disease, interviewed seven men 2 years after a myocardial infarction to describe how they created new life-styles. Larsen (1984) in Denmark also examined postmyocardial patients in a study using a longitudinal exploratory design and discovered that, for the 98 subjects, anxiety and a lack of energy were the most common problems. Graydon (1988) of Canada interviewed 79 cancer patients both prior to and after radiation treatments and found that emotional distress was a key factor affecting functional ability. In Sweden, Lundman, Asplund, and Norberg (1988) studied the problem of tedium among 158 randomly selected insulin-dependent diabetic patients and found that a higher number of women, those with higher levels of education, and those who lived alone were more likely to express their difficulties with diabetic management. Exploratory studies like these that address health problems and needs in vulnerable populations and provide answers to fundamental questions are foundational for future hypothesis-testing research.

A number of other noteworthy descriptive studies also have been focused on the aged and institutionalized. For example, Jimenez, Perez, Prieto, and Navia-Osorio (1989) studied the elderly in Spain using 207 citizens age 65 or older in nursing homes, hospitals, and at home and found that eating well, taking walks, and sleeping soundly are inversely related to depression and anxiety. In Norway, Gjertsen (1984) interviewed 500 aged individuals and measured their functional capability and social support. She found that the aged who had strong social networks were less likely to be institutionalized.

Runciman (1989) of England studied the opinions of health care providers about visiting the elderly at home. Armstrong-Esther and Browne (1986) examined nurse–patient interactions in a geriatric hospital ward and found that nurses interacted more frequently with lucid patients and gave more physical than restorative care. These studies suggested that new programs and approaches to assist the elderly in maintaining their independence are needed to improve quality of life. This research also directs attention to the nature and quality of nurses' care-giving activities.

Mothers and children, another vulnerable population, were addressed in about one-third of the clinical studies. Bayik (1984) studied contraception and abortion, using a stratified random sample of 325 Turkish women and found that induced abortions were usually sought because of economic hardship. In Australia, Fahy and Holschier (1988) examined the factors affecting the success of breastfeeding among 100 women. Zahr, Khoury, and Nugent (1988) studied 68 Lebanese infants to determine the effects of turmoil from the shelling and gunfire of civil war on physical functioning. In the Philippines, a considerable amount of significant work has been conducted on child development and the problem of malnutrition, widespread in most developing countries, by Williams and colleagues (Williams & Williams, 1989; Williams, Williams, & Dial, 1986; Williams, Williams, & Landa, 1989). Other useful assessment and intervention studies include the research on the time awareness of Japanese patients by Nojima, Oda, Nishil, Fukui, Seo, and Akiyoshi (1987), and a study of the activity needs of hospitalized surgical patients in Poland by Gorajek-Jozwik (1989).

Although many of the studies that were reviewed were focused on some aspect of health promotion, comparatively few investigators attempted to link health needs with interventions and results measured in terms of health status and provision of service factors such as the organization of care delivery, personnel, or cost. However, Candy (1987) described the use of inexpensive oral rehydration therapy for dehydrated children. In Belgium, Maas (1984) described three treatment regimens for neonate's umbilical care. Roe (1989) in England interviewed 106 nurses to determine the single best method of bladder washouts and then developed a protocol for bladder care based on the findings. Hase and Douglas (1987) of Australia, in a quasi-experimental study, determined the effect of a relaxation intervention.

Studies of how to educate clients include the one by Webb (1986), who examined the knowledge of women having hysterectomies. In the Philippines, Williams et al. (1988) conducted a study of women who underwent a mastectomy or hysterectomy and found that those who were given pre-operative instruction performed postoperative tasks at a significantly higher level. In Lebanon, Zahr, Yazigi, and Armenian (1989) examined the effect of patient education on compliance for mothers and children needing follow-up care. Jinadu, Olusi, Alade, and Ominiyi (1988) conducted a longitudinal study in Nigeria of 184 mothers with children under 5 years of age suffering from episodes of diarrhea. In this study, noteworthy because of its high social significance, the investigators found that with instruction and return demonstration, the mothers' knowledge of how to prepare oral rehydration therapy increased significantly and the children's starvation decreased.

Other notable studies focusing on the impact of training interventions on patient outcomes include the one by Hentinen (1986) in Finland. This investigator did a longitudinal analysis of 60 myocardial infarction patients and found that patient information improved the participants' knowledge of their illness and health care. Thompson (1989) studied men who had had a myocardial infarction. Subjects were randomly assigned to a patient education or a control group. Those who were given a training intervention had significantly less anxiety. Milne, Joachim, and Niedhardt (1986) conducted a longitudinal study by randomly assigning 80 patients with inflammatory bowel disease to a relaxation or control group. These researchers found that learning relaxation strategies resulted in a decrease of disease activity and stress. Mogan, Wells, and Robertson (1985) of Canada used an experimental design and randomly assigned 72 patients undergoing elective abdominal surgery to a relaxation or a control group. Those in the experimental group experienced less distress and spent more time ambulating. In summary, although some of the stronger intervention and client education studies have linked health problems and needs with interventions and changes in health status, generally little attention has been paid to assessing the costs and benefits of the nursing interventions in terms of, for example, personnel requirements, time spent in teaching, length of hospital stay, or lost work time.

Perceptions and Attitudes of Caregivers and Clients. The World Health Organization (1988) recommended that research focused on health promotion, improved life-styles, and safe environments be undertaken. Gooding, Sloan, and Amsel's (1988) exploratory study of nearly 3,000 elderly Canadians was conducted to examine the key factors determining attitudes toward well-being. Folta and Deck (1987), in a qualitative study of 457 African women in Zimbabwe, described the women's perceptions of the tensions they experience when their children and elderly are sick and choices have to be made about the use of traditional healers, modern medical care, or prayer and prophet healing. Alade (1989) studied the perceptions and knowledge of 49 pregnant adolescents in Nigeria about contraception. Uyer (1986) of Turkey examined the perceptions of care of 100 mothers in a quasi-experimental study and found that mothers of sick children who visited an outpatient clinic and received nursing support before, during, and after the visit were better able to identify and remember treatment regimens than those who did not.

Scientific endeavors that reflect a concern with understanding the clients' view of health problems and needs are considered especially beneficial (WHO, 1988). Several other studies, in addition to those previously cited, have been focused on consumers' perceptions of health needs and of health care services. In Nigeria, Olade (1989) conducted an exploratory study to improve understanding of clients' satisfaction with the care provided in an outpatient clinic and found that nurses were generally accepted as primary health care providers. In a phenomenologic investigation, Halldorsdottir (1989) in Iceland examined the behaviors of nurses and found that nurses' caring activities improved the patients' perceptions of well-being. Lindsey, Dodd, and Chen (1985) conducted an in-depth exploratory study by interviewing 40 Taiwanese oncology patients to determine their social support networks and then compared Taiwanese and American patients. In France, Bret (1984) interviewed hospitalized urology patients prior to hospital discharge and 8 days after returning home and found that for short hospital stays new methods were necessary to provide patients with take-home educational materials. In England, Teasdale (1987), using a grounded theory approach, interviewed 21 patients in a psychiatric day clinic and found that one of their greatest fears was being labeled as "mad."

In landmark research with obvious health policy implications, Norberg of Sweden and colleagues (Norberg, Asplund, & Waxman, 1987; Norberg, Backstrom, Athlin, & Norberg, 1988; Norberg & Hirschfeld, 1987) conducted a number of studies in nursing homes addressing questions related to forced feedings and withholding food (Akerlund & Norberg, 1985; Asplund & Norberg, 1984; Michaelsson, Norberg, & Samuelsson, 1987). Development of improved public policy through community participation aimed at meeting the health care needs of all citizens has been identified by the World Health Organization (1988) as a major theme for future scientific initiatives. Therefore, research with clear health policy implications or studies that reflect nurses' understanding of policy research and policymaking in local, national, and international communities were judged as especially beneficial. At the present stage of nursing science, relatively few clinical nursing studies have clear-cut implications for changes in national health policy. This is the case, too, for much of the research focused on nursing education and administration. However, there are notable exceptions. Examples of research with strong policy implications include the work cited by Williams and colleagues, Norberg and colleagues, and the exploratory research by Hirschfeld (1989), and Krulik, Hirschfeld, and Sharon (1984) describing families of impaired adults and children and the accompanying strenuous physical activity and lack of predictability.

Evaluation of the Quality of Care. As the cost of health care increases, difficult policy choices about how much care, of what type and quality, and care at what cost have to be made. Professional accountability involves participation in decisions related to setting the standards required to judge quality. One way to evaluate quality for informed decision making is to assess consumer satisfaction with the outcomes of care, with physical facilities and equipment, and with caregivers. A number of quality care evaluation studies were found in which these factors were a major focus. For example, Field (1987) examined mothers' satisfaction with labor and delivery in traditional and birth-room settings. In a study notable for its large sample size, Moores and Thompson (1986) surveyed over 1,300 patients discharged from hospitals to determine their satisfaction with the quality of the hospital facilities, personnel, and care. In Scotland, Watson (1989) performed a quasi-experimental study to examine the effectiveness of two types of urinary sheath systems, and Roe, Reid, and Brocklehurst (1988) compared four urinary drainage systems for acceptability, ease of use, and patient comfort. Assessing caregivers in Sierra Leone, Edwards (1987) conducted a study using two villages to evaluate health units and traditional birth attendants. Moyer (1989) interviewed 160 parents of children to improve understanding of the quality of the services provided by nurse specialists.

Nursing Education Research

The problems in the 134 nursing education studies pertained to student characteristics, educational programs and evaluation, or educator characteristics. The context of interest in roughly three-quarters of the studies was basic, post-basic, or university nursing education and for one-quarter it was continuing education. Nearly two-thirds of the studies were descriptive, one-quarter were program evaluations, and the remaining were methodologic. Three-fourths were cross-sectional. In nearly 100 studies, nursing students were the population of interest and in 36, educators were. Convenience samples were described most often but in many studies the sampling model was not described and random sampling was reported only rarely.

Nursing Student Characteristics. To achieve the goal of health for all, nursing students and graduates are needed whose attitudes and behaviors are as diverse as those of the people they serve. Effective health care requires nurses with a range of values, interests, and competencies to provide the appropriate kind of care to critically and chronically sick at home and in hospitals and for educating people about healthy life-styles. Well-prepared nurses are also required who can organize, manage, and supervise auxiliaries, conduct research, and provide leadership by participating in planning and implementing national health activities (WHA, 1989). Data on the characteristics of students are useful in manpower planning and policymaking and in reorientating educational programs to primary health care. To develop a demographic database in Nigeria, of the people being recruited into nursing, Adejunmobi (1986) collected statistics on nearly 300 randomly selected students enrolled in three basic and post-basic nursing programs. The social benefit of such a survey is judged as high for a country with the largest population in Sub-Saharan Africa but with an expenditure on education of only 1.4% of the gross national product as compared to 5% for all countries of the world (Human Development Report, 1990).

Focusing on students' attitudes and behaviors in Greece, four physicians (Vaslamatzis, Bazas, Lyketsos, & Katsouyanni, 1985) assessed the characteristics of 275 student nurses using Foulds' (1976) scales of anxiety, depression, and personality. Weller, Harrison, and Katz (1988) examined the self-image of 235 student nurses in two Israeli schools in a study with both a longitudinal and a cross-sectional component. Eriksson (1989) assessed the caring paradigms of 63 graduate students in the Swedish School of Nursing in Helsinki, Finland. In Canada, Gupta, McMahon, and Sandhu (1986) described health and life-styles in their examination of health risk factors for undergraduates, and Elkind (1988) described nurses' smoking behaviors. A small study concerning AIDS was reported by Bowd and Loos (1987). These Canadian researchers, using a 20-item questionnaire to describe 114 nursing students' knowledge and opinions of AIDS, found respondents reasonably well-informed. Krohwinkel (1985) in Germany described students' caregiving behaviors, and Lerheim (1985) described Norwegian students' attitudes, motivations, and feelings about nursing. The more difficult characteristics to assess, those associated with professional performance, were examined in the relatively few studies of nurses' adjustment to initial employment and their career paths (Bircumshaw & Chapman, 1988; Howard & Brooking, 1987; Reid, Nellis, & Boore, 1987).

Education Programs and Program Evaluation. Fourteen studies were reviewed that were focused primarily on nursing curriculums. In *Development of Indicators for Monitoring Progress Towards Health for All by the Year 2000* (WHO, 1981), one of the criteria considered valid for judging a country's progress in health care is the number of schools that have revised their curriculums by adapting them to primary health care. In 1985, Ohlson and Franklin emphasized population-based nursing education and the importance of the management component in nursing programs. Later in the decade, the World Health Assembly (1989) urged member states to support nurses' training in research methodology and management in order to increase the leadership of nurses in reorienting health research, nursing education, and practice for health-for-all strategies. An exemplary educational program that seems to meet these criteria is the one at the University of Kuopio, Finland. Sinkkonen (1988) described master's and doctoral study for practice, education, and administration with an emphasis on national health policy. The program is designed to overcome the limitations of single-discipline educational units; faculty are doctorally prepared in the fields of nursing, public health, and management. Other systems of education oriented toward primary health care that are cited as exemplary (WHO, 1988) include the one at Maastricht in the Netherlands and the Biomedical Science Institute in Oporto, Portugal. Research is being integrated into the curriculum, as described by Hunt (1987) in England, through action research projects: In a program that sounds extremely creative, nurse educators and managers identify problems in practice and then evaluate pertinent research and change practice accordingly. Stephenson (1985) described a research-based method for selecting curriculum content using nurses' opinions of the relevance of learning objectives. Roberts (1985) discussed the use of nursing theories to structure curriculums.

Program evaluation in the review was broadly construed to include evaluations of outcomes using scientific methods to measure single courses, training interventions, and total programs. The strongest program evaluations are useful, feasible, fair, and technically adequate (Rutman, 1984). These were the criteria we used to assess the evaluation studies. As noted, evaluations were reported in about one-quarter of the nursing education research. The World Health Organization (1979) supports evaluation research for improved understanding of the cost and benefits of education and practice. Reid (1985), at the University of Ulster, concerned about the assignment by nurse administrators of a high number of nursing students to hospital wards, evaluated the clinical learning environments, including student supervision, over 4 years. This is a timely study with relevant implications for manpower planning. According to the author, in Northern Ireland there is a sufficient number of nurses but the distribution, as for many countries, is inequitable, with the majority of the educational programs located in large urban centers, leaving outlying areas underserved. Myrick and Awrey (1988), addressing a similar theme, evaluated the differences in the clinical competencies of baccalaureate students who had preceptors and those who did not. Sohn (1986) examined the education content in 54 Canadian baccalaureate and college diploma programs and found that the general education content was overshadowed by the professional, especially in diploma programs, and that leadership was emphasized primarily at the baccalaureate level. A variety of small programs and courses have been evaluated with reasonably strong technical analyses, including those described by Coates and Chambers (1989) of an introductory 3-week computer course and another of a post-basic psychiatric nursing course by Chambers (1988).

Nurse Educator Characteristics. In a cross-national exploratory study using seven schools in the United States and Canada, Morgan (1987) analyzed the characteristics of clinical nurse teachers using the Nursing Clinical Teacher Effectiveness Inventory developed for the study. Nurses as teachers were also described by Jones (1985) and by Kanitsaki and Sellick (1989). As nurse educators develop their skills to use more complex methodologies and work collaboratively in research teams with experts in a variety of fields, more studies of a higher quality are anticipated for nursing education. The collaboration reported by Chick and Paull (1988) may prove useful in this regard. Relatively few research projects were conducted with interdisciplinary teams, and many of the evaluations appear to be short-term monitoring exercises for single events. Program evaluations of the future, where feasible, will include protocols addressing community need, resource availability, and analytic frameworks for the measurement of student and faculty performance and its outcome.

Nursing Administration Research

The two main themes of the problems for the 74 studies focused on nursing administration were human resource management and delivery of health care. The management of human resources (or manpower*) research included studies of job satisfaction, staffing and scheduling, recruitment and retention, nurse manager characteristics, and work-related stress. A significant finding was that none of the nursing administration studies were cost-benefit or cost-effectiveness analyses and few were studies involving assessments of consumer satisfaction. The hospital was the setting for more than half the research, with community and long-term care agencies accounting for only about 15 studies. Roughly three-fourths of the studies were exploratory-descriptive. Eight were program evaluations. The few remaining were quasi-experimental projects, and one was a historical analysis.

Human Resource Management. An example of the more than 50 explorative studies in this category was the one by Canadians, Cairns and Craig (1987), who gathered information about the satisfaction of hospital staff nurses using hour-long semistructured interviews. Working with patients and families was the task that staff nurses found most satisfying, a finding that is consistent with those in the many studies of nurses' satisfaction in the United States. As with the Canadian study, the majority in the United States have described nurses in hospitals. Pilkington and Wood (1986) in Australia and Metcalf (1986) in Ireland examined nurses' job satisfaction in hospitals. In the Australian study the reliable and widely validated measure of health care workers' satisfaction developed by Stamps and Piedmont (1986) was used. Other noteworthy studies of nurses' satisfaction included the one in Finland by Perala and Hentinen (1989) examining nurses' opinions before and several months after the implementation of a primary nursing assignment system in

*The authors recognize the sexist connotation of "manpower" but use the term to conserve space.

hospitals. In Ireland, Dolan (1987) examined the relationship between burnout and job satisfaction for 90 nurses in nine Dublin hospitals using the reputable Maslach Burnout Inventory (Maslach & Jackson, 1981). Zuraikat and McCloskey (1986) conducted a nationwide survey in Jordan of more than 300 hospital nurses. Dewe (1987) of New Zealand also studied hospital nurses, but in a large-scale project involving several stages and 2,500 subjects. Among the few investigators using sites other than hospitals. Power and Sharp (1988) in England compared stress and satisfaction among nearly 200 mental handicap nurses and 24 hospice nurses. Lenartowicz (1989) of Poland conducted a creative analysis of nurses' perceptions of freedom to make decisions.

It was interesting to find that convenience samples were used slightly less often in the nursing administration studies: in about two-fifths of the studies as compared to half for the nursing education and clinical research. However, a larger portion was univariate, half as compared to about one-third for the clinical and nursing education research. In many of the studies that are not cited, the sample sizes were relatively small even for the methodologies used, and power analyses to calculate effect size were rarely reported.

Staffing and scheduling, methods of work, and working conditions are among the major factors in nursing manpower analysis models. Studies of nurses' satisfaction and stress improve understanding of working conditions and scheduling patterns, as does the research by Milne and Watkins (1986) analyzing the effects of shift rotation on nurses' coping. A study of working conditions by Todd, Reid, and Robinson (1989) in Northern Ireland is also of interest both from a manpower and a clinical care perspective. These investigators used repeated measures to examine the quality of nursing care in two hospitals on wards scheduling 8- and 12-hours shifts and found that the quality of care was lower during the 12-hour shifts. A number of researchers addressed workload and staffing levels for specific patient populations. For example, Smith and Molzahn-Scott (1986) compared care requirements in long-term geriatric and acute care units. Reid and Melaugh (1988) described the nursing care hours for more than 40 midwifery awards.

In the review, a number of projects were also found that were focused on factors related to retaining nurses in the workforce and upgrading their skill. For example, in a large study using a stratified random sample of more than 2,000 nurses in England and Wales, Thomas, Nicholl, and Williams (1988) described how nurses are able to vary their work assignments and move between the public and private sectors. Barry, Soothill, and Francis (1989) examined nurses' personnel histories to demonstrate how these could be used in manpower planning. In Australia, Fox (1987) used a self-administered questionnaire to collect data from a select sample of 175 nurses about their future employment intentions. Kabat, Tobiasz-Adamczyk, and Gawel (1986) compared the demographic, epidemiologic, and occupational determinants of absences from work for several hundred female doctors and nurses in a health service unit in Krakow, Poland. Although no studies were found in which the primary focus was cost-effectiveness analysis of nursing care, Monks (1985) addressed cost in terms of nurses' time. One final class of eight studies in the manpower category pertained to nurse manager characteristics. Representative examples addressing high priority problems include those of Morrison (1989), who described charge nurses' perceptions of themselves as caregivers; Whelan (1988), who analyzed the management styles of ward sisters and related these to quality of care; and Irurita (1988), who examined the leader effectiveness of Australian head nurses.

Delivery of Health Care. Slightly more than one-third of the nursing administration research was focused on organizing and delivering health care. The problems studied were related to selecting nursing models for practice; organizational cultures and environments; assignment patterns, including primary and team nursing; delegation and the use of nonprofessionals; and new or expanded systems of health care delivery. No studies were found that primarily addressed information systems. The World Health Organization (1988) recommended that studies be conducted to improve understanding of cooperation between providers and communities. It was encouraging, therefore, to find Barbee's (1987) qualitative analysis of nurses' brokerage function between providers in traditional and modern health systems in Botswana communities. Swanson (1988), in an observational study in Cuba, described changes in people's health status and the key role of nurses in primary health care systems. The longitudinal perspective Swanson brought to her analysis, by describing health care before and after the 1959 Cuban Revolution, was especially informative. Using a high priority population of new mothers, Berry and Metcalf (1986) addressed the problem of organizing patient as opposed to talk-centered approaches for British maternity services. As part of the methodology, patient satisfaction data were collected using questionnaires and interviews.

The use of organizational theory also is encouraged by the World Health Organization in research for health care delivery (WHO, 1988). Kinnunen (1988) of Finland, relying on some of the most reputable organization science, addressed the problem of how organizational culture affects the use of scientific knowledge in practice. Milne (1986) evaluated patients' and nurses' perceptions of the milieu of psychiatric wards in a systematic evaluation project with a strong theoretical base.

Primary and team nursing were compared by a number of authors. Two Canadians, Wilson and Dawson (1989), conducted an impressive 2-year longitudinal evaluation of the assignment patterns in a geriatric long-term setting. Using Qualpacs (Wandelt & Ager, 1974) and Phaneuf's (1976) schedule for retrospective audits to assess the quality of care, Reed (1988) compared nurses' behavior and job satisfaction for primary and team nursing. However, little discussion was included about the many confounding factors. In a program evaluation, Betts (1987) assessed the extent to which having nurse aids employed in a community enabled the elderly to remain independent. This project was noteworthy because it focused simultaneously on the aged, communities, costs, and delegation of responsibility to auxiliary personnel, all factors of high priority.

New and expanded health care delivery systems was the theme of the final group of studies. A noteworthy effort was reported by Steward (1985); the establishment in the Canadian province of New Brunswick of an Extra-Mural Hospital. The institution is called a "hospital without walls" because it provides a wide range of hospital services in the homes of people living in rural localities. Jowett and Armitage (1988) reported an informative study of liaison nurses in Wales, who enhanced the continuity of care for people between hospital and home. The health care delivery research reflects investigators' concerns with more than only providers. In some studies, the recipients of care were sources of data and this is a strengh. However, it was disappointing not finding more studies of primary health care services.

SUMMARY AND FUTURE DIRECTIONS

The clinical nursing research that was reviewed provides a foundation for future study. There is a substantial amount of information describing perceptions and attitudes. However, few studies were found that examined safe environments and life-styles to improve understanding of the most appropriate interventions, especially those designed to decrease the prevalence in many countries of communicable diseases. Strong programs of research are needed that focus on the care and services for people with infectious diseases, including AIDS, and on damaging life-styles. Few studies were found addressing alcohol and substance abuse. Other factors such as safety hazards in the home and workplace, improper food preparation, polluted environments, and hazardous wastes need study to improve understanding of the health policy requirements. As new patterns of morbidity emerge, chronic disorders are diagnosed, and populations age, local health and support services will be needed to assist with the social integration of people at home, in hospitals, and in communities. Epidemiologic analyses of the patterns of health changes and the use of health services are pivotal in identifying the primary health services that are easily accessed and used especially by women, children, the elderly, the mentally disturbed, and the chronically ill or disabled.

A framework suggested by WHO (1988) for analyzing problems, which may be useful in the future, is, first, to select a high priority research problem and study the impact on the health and welfare of the most vulnerable populations; second, to employ sound empirical measures; third, to synthesize the results and make recommendations for implementation; and, fourth, to disseminate the results to policymakers and practitioners. By building on existing clinical reserch designed to improve the health status of people at a reasonable cost, leading scientists from many countries can participate in conducting the national and cross-national policy studies that are widely needed. Many of the clinical studies reviewed were judged as providing an attractive opportunity for future international collaboration. Leading nurse scientists are conducting highly significant research, including comparative studies, that are advancing theoretical understanding of health needs, care, and outcomes.

It is generally held that there are three major stages in scientific research and that each is meritorious in its own right. First, there is perception of a problem and the search for new phenomena. Second, systematic analysis to understand cause and effect takes place. Third, theories and models are developed and tested (Dutton & Crowe, 1988). Nursing research in most countries is largely first-stage science. Many studies are explorative-descriptive projects designed to identify problems, develop concepts, and generate hypotheses. In view of the evolution of nursing science, first-stage research is appropriate. The potential of a number of studies for new understanding of health and illness and the accompanying care requirements is high. This is especially the case where research programs involving a number of nurse scientists, from a number of countries, are focused on the health care needs of vulnerable populations.

Cross-national, interdisciplinary collaboration is essential to identify healthy life-style indicators that have global implications for the public and for providers. As international travel becomes commonplace and as computer technologies improve understanding of worldwide events, more collaboration about problems of pandemic proportions is anticipated. Development in the future of international classification and coding schemes of healthy life-style indicators, nursing activities, and management problems could assist with cross-national comparisons of health care outcomes. Comparative international research is also needed to describe educational programs in developing and industrialized nations. A great deal can be learned, for example, from Italy, where some nurses are working to integrate nursing education into mainstream higher education (Sansoni, 1990). Holding constant select social and economic indicators such as population size, national income, education expenditures, and school enrollment, then analyzing similarities and differences could provide useful information about alternative ways of conceiving of changes in nursing education. Or perhaps a more useful initial effort would be to assemble a series of case studies of nursing education programs like those by Katz and Fulop (1978). Yamba (1990) provided an excellent description of the primary health care component in Zambian nursing education, and Choongo (1990) discussed the organization of primary health care and nurses' leadership.

Strong programs of education and research can enhance nurses' leadership in organizing, managing, and evaluating health care services. Future study is needed to address disease and health needs and the planning, organization, management, and evaluation of effective health care services. Study is also needed of nurses' delegation of authority and responsibility and their supervision of auxiliary workers in hospitals and communities. Case studies of accomplished nurse administrators could improve understanding of leadership and management effectiveness in societies at various stages of development and of nurses' contributions to the local and national health services.

In the review, a fair amount of research was found pertaining to human resource management. But some problems have received little attention. For example, studies were not found addressing alternative organizational designs, nurse managers' work technology, on-the-job management training, or nurse migration. The problems related to some of these, to work technology for example, can be complex and difficult to analyze. Building on the seminal research in this domain by Alexander and Randolph (1985), Leatt and Schneck (1981), and Mark (1985) should prove beneficial for future studies. Knowledge is needed of the relationship between health needs and the organization of care delivery systems and the effect of these on nurses' work and its results or outcomes.

Although much more research is needed addressing the problems of health care delivery, the work reported thus far is relevant and there is some evidence that organizational theories from the private and public sector are being used. A great deal more can be learned from private sector research about efficiency and cost effectiveness. Knowledge from the public service sector can greatly enhance understanding of equity and how to assess the quality of public services. The equitable distribution of health services is problematic in nearly all countries. Framing research in terms of equity theories could improve understanding of nursing manpower distribution problems and contribute to national and international health policy.

In many countries the need for nurses and the resources required to produce skilled nursing personnel are under review. National nurses' associations are contributing to the efforts required to recruit, educate, and retain nurses. To improve understanding of the nursing resource calculus, Mejia's (1987) description may be useful in the future: "Health manpower imbalance is a discrepancy between the numbers, types, functions, distribution and quality of health workers, on the one hand, and on the other, a country's needs for their services and its ability to employ, support and maintain them" (p. 16). Future research is needed that includes population-based trend analyses that begin with demographic and epidemiologic information about the health needs of the people served. Manpower studies can then more successfully address the supply and demand for nurses. Viewing nursing resources in terms of health needs and the distribution of services rather than only in terms of demand is a future challenge. Perhaps a place to begin is with studies taking a diffusion of knowledge approach. Little research was found using this method. Studies, for example, that address how the introduction and adaptation of nursing knowledge and technology from one country to another affect the equitable distribution of nurses could be beneficial for a future in which health, health needs, and health care services are better understood by providers and the public they serve.

ACKNOWLEDGMENTS

Preparation of this chapter was supported in part by the Florida League for Nursing and Sigma Theta Tau, Delta Beta Chapter, to whom we are indebted. We are appreciative, too, for the printed proceedings contributed by several participating countries in the Workgroup of European Nurse Researchers and the documents from the national nurses' associations identified in the chapter. We also gratefully acknowledge the comments on a draft of this chapter by Miriam J. Hirschfeld, Margarethe Lorensen, Virginia Ohlson, Sirkka Sinkkonen, and Kathleen Smyth.

REFERENCES

Adejunmobi, A. (1986). Socio-demographic characteristics and opinions of basic and post-basic nursing students in Nigeria. *International Journal of Nursing Studies, 23,* 337–347.

Alade, M. (1989). Teenage pregnancy in Ile-Ife, Western Nigeria. *Western Journal of Nursing Research, 11*(5), 609–613.

Alexander, J. W., & Randolph, W. A. (1985). The fit between technology and structure as a predictor of performance in nursing subunits. *Academy of Management Journal, 28,* 844–859.

Akerlund, B., & Norberg, A. (1985). An ethical analysis of double bind conflicts as experienced by care workers feeding severely demented patients. *International Journal of Nursing Studies, 22*(3), 207–216.

Armstrong-Esther, C., & Browne, K. (1986). The influence of elderly patients' mental impairment on nurse-patient interaction. *Journal of Advanced Nursing, 11,* 379–387.

Asplund, K., & Norberg, A. (1984). Caregivers' experience of the care of senile demented patients in the final stage of the disease. *Proceedings of the 7th Workgroup Meeting of the Workgroup of European Nurse-Researchers* (pp. 388–393). London, England: Royal College of Nursing.

Barbee, E. L. (1987). Tensions in the brokerage role. *Western Journal of Nursing Research, 9,* 244–256.

Barry, J. T., Soothill, K. L., & Francis, B. J. (1989). Nursing the statistics: A demonstration study of nurse turnover and retention. *Journal of Advanced Nursing, 14,* 528–535.

Bayik, A. (1984). An epidemiological study of abortion in Bornova-Izmir. *Proceedings of the 7th Workgroup Meeting of the Workgroup of European Nurse-Researchers* (pp. 306–313). London, England: Royal College of Nursing.

Berry, A. J., & Metcalf, C. L. (1986). Paradigms and practice: The organization of the delivery of nursing care. *Journal of Advanced Nursing, 11,* 589–597.

Betts, G. (1987). Evaluation of a nursing aides scheme for elderly people. *Journal of Advanced Nursing, 12,* 85–94.

Bircumshaw, D., & Chapman, C. M. (1988). A study to compare the practice style of graduate and non-graduate nurses and midwives: The pilot study. *Journal of Advanced Nursing, 13,* 605–614.

Bowd, A. D., & Loos, C. H. (1987). Nursing students' knowledge and opinions concerning AIDS. *Canadian Journal of Nursing Research, 19*(4), 11–19.

Bret, J. (1984). Specific problems of patients with trans-urethral resection of the prostate during their convalescence. *Proceedings of the 7th Workgroup Meeting of the Workgroup of European Nurse-Researchers* (pp. 535–541). London, England: Royal College of Nursing.

Candy, C. (1987). Recent advances in the care of children with acute diarrhea: Giving responsibility to the nurse and parents. *Journal of Advanced Nursing, 12,* 95–99.

Caims, B. J. S., & Cragg, C. E. (1987). Sources of job satisfaction and dissatisfaction among baccalaureate staff nurses in hospitals. *Canadian Journal of Nursing Research, 19,* 15–29.

Chambers, M. (1988). Curriculum evaluation: An approach towards appraising a post-basic psychiatric nursing course. *Journal of Advanced Nursing, 13,* 330–340.

Chick, N., & Paull, D. (1988). Collaboration between nurse educators in Australia and New Zealand extends educational opportunities for nurses. *International Journal of Nursing Studies, 25,* 279–286.

Choongo, D. E. (1990). Organization of PHC in Zambia and the nursing leadership role. *The Zambia Nurse, 15*(1), 9–12.

Choates, V. E., & Chambers, M. (1989). Teaching microcomputing to student nurses: An evaluation. *Journal of Advanced Nursing, 14,* 152–157.

Dewe, P. (1987). Identifying strategies nurses use to cope with work stress. *Journal of Advanced Nursing, 12,* 489–497.

Dolan, N. (1987). The relationship between burnout and job satisfaction in nurses. *Journal of Advanced Nursing, 12,* 3–12.

Dutton, J. A., & Crowe, L. (1988). Setting priorities among scientific initiatives. *American Scientist, 76,* 599–603.

Edwards, N. (1987). Traditional birth attendants in Sierra Leone: Key providers of maternal and child health care in West Africa. *Western Journal of Nursing Research, 9*(3), 335–347.

Elkind, A. K. (1988). The effect of training on knowledge and opinion about smoking amongst nurses and student teachers. *Journal of Advanced Nursing, 13,* 57–69.

Eriksson, K. (1989). Caring paradigms. *Scandinavian Journal of Caring Sciences, 3,* 169–176.

Fahy, K., & Holschier, J. (1988). Success or failure with breast feedings. *Australian Journal of Advanced Nursing, 5*(3), 12–18.

Field, P. (1987). Maternity nurses: How parents see us. *International Journal of Nursing Studies, 24*(3), 191–199.

Folta, J., & Deck, E. (1987). Rural Zimbabwean Shona women: Illness concepts and behavior. *Western Journal of Nursing Research, 9*(3), 301–316.

Ford, J. (1989). Living with a history of a heart attack: A human science investigation. *Journal of Advanced Nursing, 14,* 173–179.

Foulds, G. A. (1976). *The hierarchical nature of personal illness.* London: Academic Press.

Fox, S. (1987). The origins of wastage from nursing. *Australian Journal of Advanced Nursing, 5*(1), 11–17.

Gjertsen, E. (1984). Self-care ability and functional capacity of elderly people in the municipality of Bergen, Norway. *Proceedings of the Workgroup Meeting of the Workgroup of European Nurse-Researchers* (pp. 436–446). London, England: Royal College of Nursing.

Gooding, B., Sloan, M., & Amsel, R. (1988). The well-being of older Canadians. *The Canadian Journal of Nursing Research, 20*(2), 5–18.

Gorajek-Jozwik, J. (1989). The level and structure of day activity of surgical patients. *Proceedings of the 12th Workgroup Meeting and International Nursing Research Conference, Workgroup of European Nurse Researchers* (pp. 334–344). Frankfurt, Germany: German Nursing Association.

Graydon, J. (1988). Factors that predict patients' functioning following treatment for cancer. *International Journal of Nursing Studies, 25*(2), 227–324.

Gupta, A., McMahon, S., & Sandhu, G. (1986). Identification of health risk factors among undergraduate university students. *Canadian Journal of Nursing Research, 18*(2), 25–30.

Halldorsdottir, S. (1989). The essential structure of a caring and an uncaring encounter with a nurse: The patient's perspective. *Proceedings of the 12th Workgroup Meeting and International Nursing Research Conference, Workgroup of European Nurse Researchers* (pp. 309–333). Frankfurt, Germany: German Nursing Association.

Hankins, C. A. (1990). A research agenda for the 1990s. *World Health,* November–December, 24–26.

Hase, G., & Douglas, A. (1987). Effects of relaxation training on recovery from myocardial infarction. *Australian Journal of Advanced Nursing, 5*(1), 18–27.

Hentinen, M. (1986). Teaching and adaptation of patients with myocardial infarction. *International Journal of Nursing Studies, 23*(2), 125–138.

Hirschfeld, M. J. (1989). Nursing research and community nursing—The work of family care. *Proceedings of the 12th Workgroup Meeting and International Nursing Research Conference, Workgroup of European Nurse Researchers* (pp. 119–133). Frankfurt, Germany: German Nursing Association.

Holleran, C. (1988). Nursing beyond national boundaries: The 21st century. *Nursing Outlook, 36*(2), 72–75.

Howard, J. M., & Brooking, J. I. (1987). The career paths of nursing graduates from Chelsea College, University of London. *International Journal of Nursing Studies, 24,* 181–189.

Human Development Report 1990. (1990). United Nations Development Programme: Oxford, England: Oxford University Press.

Hunt, M. (1987). The process of translating research findings into nursing practice. *Journal of Advanced Nursing, 12,* 101–110.

Irurita, V. (1988). A study of nurse leadership. *Australian Journal of Advanced Nursing, 6*(1), 43–51.

Jimenez, C., Perez, T., Prieto, F., & Navia-Osorio, P. (1989). Behavioral habits and affective disorders in old people. *Journal of Advanced Nursing, 14,* 356–364.

Jinadu, M., Olusi, S., Alade, O., & Ominiyi, C. (1988). Effectiveness of primary health-care nurses in the promotion of oral rehydration therapy in a rural area in Nigeria. *International Journal of Nursing Studies, 25*(3), 185–190.

Jones, J. A. (1985). A study of nurse tutors' conceptualization of their ward teaching role. *Journal of Advanced Nursing, 10,* 349–360.

Jowett, S., & Armitage, S. (1988). Hospital and community liaison links in nursing: The role of the liaison nurse. *Journal of Advanced Nursing, 13,* 589–597.

Kabat, Z., Tobiasz-Adamczyk, B., & Gawel, G. (1986). Sickness absences of nurses and female doctors in Poland. *International Nursing Review, 33*(6), 183–185.

Kanitsaki, O., & Sellick, K. (1989). Clinical nurse teaching: An investigation of student perceptions of clinical nurse teacher behaviors. *Australian Journal of Advanced Nursing, 6*(4), 18–24.

Katz, F. M., & Fulop, T. (1978). *Personnel for health care: Case studies of educational programmes.* World Health Organization: Geneva, Switzerland.

Kinnunen, J. (1988). Impact of organizational culture on use of scientific knowledge in nursing practice. *Scandinavian Journal of Caring Sciences, 2,* 123–128.

Krohwinkel, M. (1985). Illuminating nursing practice as a contribution towards education development. *Proceedings of the 12th Workgroup Meeting and International Nursing Research Conference, Workgroup of European Nurse Researchers* (pp. 63–78) Frankfurt, Germany: German Nursing Association.

Krulik, T., Hirschfeld, M. J., & Sharon, R. (1984). Family care for the severely handicapped children and aged in Israel. Monograph, Department of Nursing, Sackler School of Medicine, Tel Aviv University, Israel.

Larsen, H. (1984). Rehabilitation after cardiac infarct. *Proceedings of the 7th Workgroup Meeting of the Workgroup of European Nurse-Researchers* (pp. 555–559). London, England: Royal College of Nursing.

Leatt, P., & Schneck, R. (1981). Nursing subunit technology: A replication. *Administrative Science Quarterly, 26,* 225–286.

Lenartowicz, H. (1989). Perceptions of nurses' freedom of making decisions at work. *Proceedings of the 12th Workgroup Meeting and International Nursing Research Conference, Workgroup of European Nurse Researchers* (pp. 408–412). Frankfurt, Germany: German Nursing Association.

Lerheim, K. (1985). Nursing education and student reactions. *Proceedings of the 12th Workgroup Meeting and International Nursing Research Conference, Workgroup of European Nurse Researchers* (pp. 100–108). Frankfurt, Germany: German Nursing Association.

Lindsey, A., Dodd, M., & Chen, S.-G. (1985). Social support network of Taiwanese cancer patients. *International Journal of Nursing Studies, 22*(2), 249–264.

Lundman, B., Asplund, K., & Norberg, A. (1988). Tedium among patients with insulin-dependent diabetes mellitus. *Journal of Advanced Nursing, 13,* 23–31.

Maas, A. (1984). Evaluation of three umbilical cord-care procedures in normal newborns. *Proceedings of the 7th Workgroup Meeting of the Workgroup of European Nurse-Researchers* (pp. 289–305). London, England: Royal College of Nursing.

Mark, B. (1985). Task and structural correlates of organizational effectiveness in private psychiatric hospitals. *Health Services Research, 20,* 199–224.

Maslach, C., & Jackson, S. E. (1981). *Maslach burnout inventory manual.* Palo Alto, CA: Consulting Psychologist Press.

Mejia, A. (1987). The nature of the challenge. In Z. Bankowski & T. Fulop (Eds.), *Health manpower out of balance* (pp. 15–40). Geneva, Switzerland: Council of International Organizations of Medical Sciences.

Metcalf, C. A. (1986). Job satisfaction and organizational change in a maternity hospital. *International Journal of Nursing Studies, 23,* 285–298.

Michaelsson, E., Norberg, A., & Samuelsson, S.-M. (1987). Assessment of thirst among severely demented patients in the terminal phase of life. Exploratory interviews with ward sisters and enrolled nurses. *International Journal of Nursing Studies, 24*(2), 87–93.

Milne, B., Joachim, G., & Niedhardt, J. (1986). A stress management programme for inflammatory bowel disease patients. *Journal of Advanced Nursing, 11,* 561–567.

Milne, D. (1986). Planning and evaluating innovations in nursing practice by measuring the ward atmosphere. *Journal of Advanced Nursing, 11,* 203–210.

Milne, D., & Watkins, F. (1986). An evaluation of the effects of shift rotation on nurses' stress, coping and strain. *International Journal of Nursing Studies, 23,* 139–146.

Mogan, J., Wells, N., & Robertson, E. (1985). Effects of preoperative teaching on postoperative pain: A replication and expansion. *International Journal of Nursing Studies, 22*(3), 267–280.

Monks, J. (1985). Reflections on the cost of hospital nursing: A comparison of factors affecting time distribution in ward, theatre, and outpatient departments. *Journal of Advanced Nursing, 10,* 103–110.

Moores, B., & Thompson, A. (1986). What 1357 hospital inpatients think about aspects of their stay in British acute hospitals. *Journal of Advanced Nursing, 11,* 87–102.

Morgan, J. (1987). Characteristics of 'best' and 'worst' clinical teachers as perceived by university nursing faculty and students. *Journal of Advanced Nursing, 12,* 331–337.

Morrison, P. (1989). Nursing and caring: A personal construct theory study of some nurses' self-perceptions. *Journal of Advanced Nursing, 14,* 421–426.

Moyer, A. (1989). Caring for a child with diabetes: The effect of specialist nurse care on parents' needs and concerns. *Journal of Advanced Nursing, 14,* 536–545.

Myrick, F., & Awrey, J. (1988). The effect of preceptorship on the clinical competency of baccalaureate student nurses: A pilot study. *Canadian Journal of Nursing Research, 20*(3), 29–43.

Nojima, Y., Oda, A., Nishil, H., Fukui, M., Seo, K., & Akiyoshi, H. (1987).

Perception of time among Japanese inpatients. *Western Journal of Nursing Research, 9*(3), 288–300.
Norberg, A., Asplund, K., & Waxman, H. (1987). Withdrawing feeding and withholding artificial nutrition from severely demented patients: Interview with caregivers. *Western Journal of Nursing Research, 9*(3), 348–356.
Norberg, A., Backstrom, A., Athlin, E., & Norberg, B. (1988). Food refusal amongst nursing home patients as conceptualized by nurses aids and enrolled nurses: An interview study. *Journal of Advanced Nursing, 13,* 478–483.
Norberg, A., & Hirschfeld, M. (1987). Feeding of severely demented patients in institutions: Interviews with caregivers in Israel. *Journal of Advanced Nursing, 12,* 551–557.
Ohlson, V. M., & Franklin, M. (1985). *An international perspective on nursing practice* (Report No. 68F 2M). Kansas City, MO: American Nurses' Association.
Olade, R. (1989). Perception of nurses in expanded roles. *International Journal of Nursing Studies, 26*(1), 15–25.
Perala, M., & Hentinen, M. (1989). Primary nursing: Opinions of nursing staff before and during implementation. *International Journal of Nursing Studies, 26,* 231–242.
Phaneuf, M. (1976). *The nursing audit.* Norwalk, CT: Appleton-Century-Crofts.
Pilkington, W., & Wood, J. (1986). Job satisfaction, role conflict and role ambiguity—a study of hospital nurses. *Australian Journal of Advanced Nursing, 3*(3), 3–14.
Power, K. G., & Sharp, G. R. (1988). A comparison of sources of nursing stress and job satisfaction among mental handicap and hospice nursing staff. *Journal of Advanced Nursing, 13,* 726–732.
Reed, S. (1988). A comparison of nurse-related behavior, philosophy of care and job satisfaction in team and primary nursing. *Journal of Advanced Nursing, 13,* 383–395.
Reid, N. G. (1985). The effective training of nurses: Manpower implications. *International Journal of Nursing Studies, 22,* 89–98.
Reid, N. G., Nellis, P., & Boore, J. (1987). Graduate nurses in Northern Ireland: Their career paths, aspirations and problems. *International Journal of Nursing Studies, 24,* 215–225.
Reid, N. G., & Melaugh, M. (1988). Nurse hours per patients: A method for monitoring and explaining staffing levels. *International Journal of Nursing Studies, 24*(1), 1–14.
Roberts, K. L. (1985). Conceptual frameworks and the nursing curriculum. *Journal of Advanced Nursing, 10,* 43–49.
Roe, B., (1989). Use of bladder washouts: A study of nurses' recommendations. *Journal of Advanced Nursing, 14,* 494–500.
Roe, B., Reid, F., & Brocklehurst, J. (1988). Comparison of four urine drainage systems. *Journal of Advanced Nursing, 13,* 374–382.
Runciman, P. (1989). Health assessment of the elderly at home: The case for shared learning. *Journal of Advanced Nursing, 14,* 111–119.
Rutman, L. (1984). *Evaluation research methods: A basic guide.* Newbury Park, CA: Sage.
Sansoni, J. (1990). *Nursing education in Italy: Reality and prospects.* Unpublished manuscript, University of Rome, Institute of Health, Rome, Italy.
Scheuch, E. K. (1990). The development of comparative research: Towards causal

explanations. In E. Oyen (Ed.), *Comparative methodology* (pp. 18–37). London: Sage.

Sinkkonen, S. (1988). University education in caring sciences in Finland. *Scandinavian Journal of Caring Sciences, 2,* 51–57.

Sivard, R. L. (1989). *World military and social expenditures.* Washington, DC: World Priorities.

Smith, D. L., & Molzahn-Scott, A. E. (1986). A comparison of nursing care requirements of patients in long-term geriatric and acute care nursing units. *Journal of Advanced Nursing, 11,* 315–321.

Sohn, K. S. (1986). General education in nursing: Current practices and faculty attitudes. *Canadian Journal of Nursing Research, 18*(4), 41–56.

Stamps, P., & Piedmont, E. (1986). *Nurses and work satisfaction.* Lexington, MA: D. C. Heath.

Stephenson, P. M. (1985). A research-based method of selecting curriculum content. *Journal of Advanced Nursing, 10,* 3–13.

Steward, J. (1985). Hospitals without walls: The New Brunswick extra-mural hospital. *International Nursing Review, 33,* 181–183.

Swanson, J. M. (1988). Health-care delivery in Cuba: Nursing's roles in achievement of the goal of 'Health for all'. *International Journal of Nursing Studies, 25,* 11–21.

Teasdale, K. (1987). Stigma and psychiatric day care. *Journal of Advanced Nursing, 12,* 339–346.

Teune, H. (1990). Comparing countries: Lessons learned. In E. Oyen (Ed.), *Comparative methodology* (pp. 38–62). London: Sage.

Thomas, K. J., Nicholl, J. P., & Williams, B. T. (1988). A study of the movement of nurses and nursing skills between the NHS and the private sector in England and Wales. *International Journal of Nursing Studies, 25,* 1–10.

Thompson, D. (1989). A randomized controlled trial of in-hospital nursing support for first time myocardial infarction patients and their partners: Effects on anxiety and depression. *Journal of Advanced Nursing, 14,* 291–297.

Todd, C., Reid, N., & Robinson, G. (1989). The quality of nursing care on wards working eight and twelve hour shifts: A repeated measures study using the MONITOR index of quality care. *International Journal of Nursing Studies, 26,* 359–368.

Uyer, G. (1986). Effect of nursing approach in understanding physicians' directions, by the mothers of sick children in an out-patient clinic. *International Journal of Nursing Studies, 23*(1), 79–85.

Vaslamatzis, G., Bazas, T., Lyketsos, G., & Katsouyanni, K. (1985). Dysthymic distress and hostile personality characteristics in Greek student nurses: A comparative study. *International Journal of Nursing Studies, 22,* 15–20.

Wandelt, M. A., & Ager, J. W. (1974). *Quality patient care scale.* Norwalk, CT: Appleton-Century-Crofts.

Watson, R. (1989). A nursing trial of urinary sheath systems on male hospitalized patients. *Journal of Advanced Nursing, 14,* 467–470.

Webb, C. (1986). Professional and lay social support for hysterectomy patients. *Journal of Advanced Nursing, 11,* 167–177.

Weller, L., Harrison, M., & Katz, Z. (1988). Changes in the self and professional images of student nurses. *Journal of Advanced Nursing, 13,* 170–184.

Whelan, J. (1988). Ward sisters' management styles and their effects on nurses' perceptions of quality of care. *Journal of Advanced Nursing, 13,* 124–138.

Williams, P., Valderrama, D., Gloria, M., Pascoguin, L., Saavedra, S., De La Rama, D., Ferry, T., Abaguin, C., & Zaldivar, S. (1988). Effects of preparation for mastectomy/hysterectomy on women's post-operative self-care behaviors. *International Journal of Nursing Studies, 25*(3), 191–206.

Williams, P., & Williams, A. (1989). Mild malnutrition and child development in the Philippines. *Western Journal of Nursing Research, 11*(3), 310–319.

Williams, P., Williams, A., & Dial, M. (1986). Children at risk: Perinatal events, developmental delays and the effects of a developmental stimulation program. *International Journal of Nursing Studies, 23*(1), 21–38.

Williams, P., Williams, A., & Landa, A. (1989). Factors influencing performance of chronically ill chicken on a developmental screening test. *International Journal of Nursing Studies, 26*(2), 163–172.

Wilson, N. M., & Dawson, P. (1989). A comparison of primary nursing and team nursing in a geriatric long-term care setting. *International Journal of Nursing Studies, 26,* 1–13.

World Health Assembly Resolution 42.27. (1989). *Strengthening nursing and midwifery in support of strategies for health for all.* Geneva, Switzerland: World Health Organization.

World Health Organization. (1979). *Evaluation of inpatient nursing practice.* Copenhagen, Denmark: World Health Organization, Regional Office for Europe.

World Health Organization. (1981). *Development of indicators for monitoring progress towards health for all by the year 2000.* Geneva, Switzerland.

World Health Organization. (1984). *Education and training of nurse teachers and managers with special regard to primary care.* Geneva, Switzerland.

World Health Organization. (1987). *Evaluation of the strategy for health for all by the year 2000.* Geneva, Switzerland.

World Health Organization. (1988). *Priority research for health for all.* Copenhagen, Denmark: World Health Organization, Regional Office for Europe.

Yamba, R. (1990). Primary health care in relation to nursing education in Zambia. *The Zambia Nurse, 15*(1), 3–7.

Zahr, L., Khoury, M., & Nugent, K. (1988). Neonatal behavior of prenatally stressed Lebanese infants. *Image, 20*(4), 200–202.

Zahr, L., Yazigi, A., & Armenian, H. (1989). The effect of education and written material on compliance of pediatric clients. *International Journal of Nursing Studies, 26*(3), 213–220.

Zuraikat, N., & McCloskey, J. (1986). Job satisfaction among Jordanian registered nurses. *International Nursing Review, 33*(5), 143–146.

Index

Contents of Previous Volumes

VOLUME I

VOLUME II

VOLUME III

VOLUME IV

VOLUME V

VOLUME VI

ORDER FORM

Save 10% on Volume 10 with this coupon.

___ Check here to order the ANNUAL REVIEW OF NURSING RESEARCH, Volume 10, 1992 at a 10% discount. You will receive an invoice requesting pre-payment.

Save 10% on all future volumes with a continuation order.

___Check here to place your continuation order for the ANNUAL REVIEW OF NURSING RESEARCH. You will receive a pre-payment invoice with a 10% discount upon publication of each new volume, beginning with Volume 10, 1992. You may pay for prompt shipment or cancel with no obligation.

Name ____

Institution ____

Address ____

City/State/Zip ____

Examination copies for possible course adoption are available to instructors "on approval" only. Write on institutional letterhead, noting course, level, present text, and expected enrollment (Include $3.00 for postage and handling). Prices slightly higher overseas. Prices subject to change.

Mail this coupon to:
SPRINGER PUBLISHING COMPANY
536 Broadway, New York, N.Y. 10012